Chronic Inflammation

The "Not so Silent" Killer

Dr . Mina Nazih Botros

First paperback edition November 2018

Book design by Dr. Mina N. Botros
Images contributed thanks to Wikimedia Commons

ISBN: 978-1-7906-6921-9

DEDICATION

This book is dedicated to my parents, my sisters, my friends, my professors and mentors who believed in me from the beginning. To all the wonderful people who have entrusted me with their health.   And of course to you, the reader, may this book be a cornerstone in transforming your health.

CONTENTS

Dr. Mina Botros

*Disclaimer:

The information and materials provided in this book are designed to provide helpful information on the subjects discussed. This book is not meant to be used, to diagnose, treat, or cure any medical condition. For diagnosis or treatment of any medical or health problem, please consult your own physician. The publisher and author are not responsible for any specific health or allergy needs that may require medical supervision and are not liable for any damages or negative consequences from any treatment, action, application or preparation, to any person reading or following the information in this book. References are provided for informational purposes only and do not constitute endorsement of any websites or other sources. Readers should be aware that the websites listed in this book may change.

PREFACE
WHY DO YOU WANT TO CHANGE YOUR LIFE?

The book you are holding in your hands has the potential to quite literally change the course of your life. The contents within have been used not only in my clinic but in many other clinics to give life to those who were once in pain, suffering, and believed that they could no longer be able to do the things that they love to do. Now, more than ever, we have a wealth of resources, information, and experts in the field of health, and yet it seems like being healthy has become more difficult than ever. Being healthy has become a completely foreign process for most of us.

But not anymore, I want to empower you with the information, tips, and advice that can potentially give you your life back. The best part is that this book is not just a book, but a system that I have created and used to produce life-changing outcomes with countless patients.

This book is the sum of materials that I have gathered through extensive research, up-to-date literature, my academic pursuits, and my clinical experience. I have compiled all that information, used, tested, and perfected it to be able to produce the best outcome for my patients. But realize, that information alone is good, but it is not enough. With a few strokes on our keyboard, we can virtually learn about any topic online. The problem isn't a "lack of information", but rather the lack of how to take that information and turn it into actionable steps. What is truly unique about this book is that through my clinical experience, I have figured out how to present important information in a way that gives you the best chance to not just learn, but do the outlined steps, so that you can obtain the life-changing health benefits you desire.

I have developed a system that will allow you to take actionable steps as soon as today so that you can begin your journey to optimal health. Some of the things outlined in this book include; the principles for developing new habits by modifying your brain's reward system so that it can work with you not against you, how to alter your cravings, the two-part health ratio that most people get wrong, what foods are contributing to our illnesses, and so much more. All I ask is that you read this with an open mind and try your best to apply the assignments given at the end of each chapter. It really is that simple. I have used the information in this book with countless patients to help them transform, recover, and heal their bodies, minds, and to lift their spirits, and I am sure that if you follow the principles outlined in this book, you too can change your life too.

To get the most out of this book, I would highly encourage you to read each chapter in order and to take the necessary actions steps outlined in each chapter. This is what has produced the best outcomes for even my most stubborn of patients and I am certain that with some patience, consistency, and an open mind you will look back on your life to this very moment, right now, and be filled with abundant gratitude and amazement at the progress you have made.

It is important to realize that the media has brainwashed us to believe that healing is just "around the corner" and that amazing results can happen overnight.

Just as most disease develops progressively over time, so too does healing take time. True healing happens naturally and it takes time. You are literally changing your biology, cellular functions, chemical mechanisms in your body, enzymes, and reducing inflammatory processes that have been there for years (and if you are like any of my patients, even decades). These things may take time.

Be sympathetic to your body, it is doing its best and it truly wants to be healed, it just needs the building blocks and the step-by-step process outlined here. If you fall off track, don't feel guilty or upset, simply pick up where you left off and continue along on your health journey. With that being said, there are many people who start noticing results as soon as one or two weeks, if that is you, you are one of the lucky ones, for the rest of us, hang in there, trust me, you will be glad that you did.

So let us start with our first assignment. From my experience, the difference between those who achieve great, lasting results and those who don't, comes down to one key factor. That is being able to clearly identify your **"why"**. Your **Why** is your reason for wanting to change your life. Most of us know that it is so much easier to keep the same old habits, eat the same foods, think the same thoughts, and do the same things that have lead us here in the first place. Chances are if you are reading this book, there is something in your health that you would like to be able to achieve. If we continue to do what we have always done, we will continue to get what we have always gotten.

Why change? **Why** now? This is a very important question because your **"why"** is the most important factor as to how resilient you will be when the temptation to go back to your old habits, thoughts, and eating patterns come back. Whenever you feel discouraged, or fall off track, or want to return to the familiarity of your old habits, read your **"whys"**. They will fuel your motivation and strengthen your willpower to be able to continue to take the proper action steps outlined in this book, to take your health to a whole new level.

This is a very important exercise, so take as long as you need to, think about them, feel them, use your imagination if you have to, and you will notice that you are even more motivated to move along in your healing journey. This is the first step, I would not recommend you move any further in this book until you have clearly identified your **"whys"**.

Why do I want to change my life? Why now?

Today's Date: _________________

1.____

2.____

3.____

4.____

5.____

Now that we have identified your **"whys"**, we can move on into the next chapter.

Let the healing begin!

THE WAKE UP CALL

WHAT DO YOU HOPE TO GAIN FROM THIS BOOK?

Whether directly or indirectly, we all have been impacted by the negative effects of heart disease, Alzheimer's, diabetes, various autoimmune diseases, arthritis, and/or obesity. And now more than ever, we have reached an all-time high for mood disorders such as depression, anxiety, and even ADHD. Have you ever wondered why these diseases have continued to rise even though we are constantly making advancements in the medical field? One thing is for certain, it is not due to lack of funding. As a matter of fact, the United States has spent hundreds of billions of dollars annually to find effective ways to treat and cure these common **"age-related"** diseases. We have been lead to believe that most of these are just a consequence of living longer. But as you are about to find out in this book, this is not necessarily true. The reality is, we have more power over our health than we think or even recognize.

Sadly, it seems like for every step forward we make in medicine, we take two steps backward. We are living longer than ever and yet our quality of life has gone down the drain. We are seeing that these so-called **"age-related diseases"** are becoming more common in younger and younger individuals. Even "adult onset diabetes" has been officially renamed "type II diabetes" because we are seeing more and more kids developing it, whereas 20 years ago, this was typically only seen in adults. It should be noted that this type of diabetes is completely preventable. It is now estimated that this new generation, will be the first generation in the history of mankind to not outlive their parents. This is a problem, and it needs to be addressed.

Chronic diseases and conditions—such as heart disease, stroke, cancer, type 2 diabetes, obesity, and arthritis—are among the most common and costly causes of death and disability in the United States. Not only do they rob us of our loved ones, but they rob us from our ability to enjoy life to the fullest, to do the things we love with the people we love. If you are not sold on the crisis that is unfolding before us, just take a look at these alarming statistics from the World Health Organization (WHO) and Center of Disease Control and Prevention (CDC):

- One in four adults has two or more chronic health conditions.
- Seven of the top 10 causes of death in 2014 were chronic diseases.
- Arthritis is the most common cause of disability. Of the 54 million adults with doctor-diagnosed arthritis, more than 23 million say they have trouble with their usual activities because of their arthritis.
- Diabetes is the leading cause of kidney failure, lower-limb amputations other than those caused by injury, and new cases of blindness among adults.

For a developed country with an abundance of resources, food, health care providers, and researchers, we really should not be seeing such staggering statistics. According to OECD, in 2017, we spend the highest percentage of our country's wealth for health care and treatments and yet we are ranked as the 43rd "healthiest" nation in the world by the World Health Organization.

We have third world countries living healthier than us. This is alarming and I think we can all agree that this is, quite frankly, unacceptable. To make matters worse, not only are these chronic diseases robing us of our health, but our medical bills were found to be the number one reason for declaring bankruptcy here in the United States. Simply put, most of us cannot afford to be sick. Hopefully by now you are starting to see the picture clearly and it is not pretty. We are literally suffering unnecessarily, dying younger, and paying more than we can afford to be healthy, and yet we have nothing to show for it. Clearly, there is something very wrong going on here and no one is really talking about it.

With all of these disturbing statistics, it can be shocking to realize that these chronic diseases are mostly preventable; this is where this book comes in. Chronic diseases are diseases that take time to develop, they don't happen overnight. The bad news is that this makes them very easy to ignore until it is usually too late. The good news, however, is that because they take time to develop, we can actually play a direct role in preventing and sometimes even reversing their detrimental development in our bodies.

I know these facts and statistics are grim, but I don't want you to lose hope, despite all of this, there is a reasonable solution. If you study all these common yet deadly "age-related" chronic diseases, you'll find that they have one thing in common, and that is **"chronic inflammation"**. That is what this book is about. What is this chronic inflammation, why is it causing all these problems, and most importantly, what can we do about it? Just by the fact that you are reading this book right now, you are ahead of most people and by implementing the advice, techniques, and methods mentioned here, you have the best opportunity to reclaim your life and help your loved ones do the same.

The greatest gift I can offer you as a practicing physician are the practical techniques, steps, and methods to reduce chronic inflammation so that you can live a healthy, vibrant, fulfilling life.

Let us dive right into your next exercise to ensure your success with this book. In the last chapter, I asked you to identify your **"whys"**. That is the fuel that will keep you going when you feel tempted to quit. It will remind you of why you picked up this book, why you have committed to changing your health, why you will not go back to your old ways. For this chapter, I am going to ask you to identify specifically **"what"** it is that you hope to achieve from this book. This is a very important step because your health journey can be likened to a road trip. Having your "whys" is like having the fuel in your car, without it, you just won't get too far. However, having a full tank of gas in your car is great, but it isn't very helpful if you don't know where you are going. The "what" is your destination. By identifying what it is that you hope to achieve from this book, you will have a road map as to whether you are heading in the right or wrong direction. If you find yourself going further and further from what you would like to achieve (your destination), then all you got to do is figure out what you are doing (or not doing) that lead you there and resume the proper course. Your "whys" are your fuel and your "whats" are your compass, just by taking the time to identify each of these aspects, you are already setting yourself up for success.

What results do you hope to achieve from reading this book?

1.____

2.____

3.____

4.____

5.____

14

INFLAMMATION
THE GOOD, THE BAD, THE UGLY

In order for us to understand how chronic inflammation has single-handedly contributed to some of the most dangerous and common diseases in the United States, we must first understand what's the function of inflammation. You see, inflammation has gotten a negative reputation, whenever we hear that word, we associate it with something bad. But that is just one aspect of inflammation, in reality, inflammation within itself is not inherently bad. As a matter of fact, inflammation is actually essential for our health and wellbeing.

Inflammation is an **immune response** that gets triggered when the body detects irritants, damaged cells, disease, and/or pathogens. When we have a healthy inflammatory response, our bodies are able to recover from illness, injuries, and effectively eliminate pathogens, toxins, and irritants.

On the surface this may seem pretty simple, however, inflammation is actually quite complex. At any given second, millions of cells in your body die, and millions more are created to replace them. This is very normal and should not be alarming or concerning. Different cells have different lifespans, and biologically speaking, seven years from now, every single cell that you have now, will have been replaced with a new one. If a cell is damaged and can be repaired, inflammation restores it back to health. If the cell dies, inflammation breaks it down and removes it so that the new cell can take its place and function.

Thus inflammation is essential for the reconstructing of damaged cells in our bodies and the removal of dead cells. An example that we can all relate to is exercise. Exercise has countless health benefits and I can write a whole book just about the positive effects exercise has on the body. But for now, I will focus on exercise and inflammation. After completing a workout for the first time, many of us can recall that severe soreness and stiffness that develops over the next two to three days. That is because, during the workout, we exerted a lot of muscular energy and pushed them more than they are used to getting worked and thus they get little micro tears, little micro damage to the muscle cells. If that is all that happened after you exercised then we would just be damaging our muscles until we have no more healthy muscle cells to be able to move. Thankfully, that is not the case.

After a workout, our body sends the appropriate inflammatory markers and begins to recover those damaged cells and actually begins to strengthen and rebuild them. The body's inflammatory response is what allows you to recover and rebuild those muscle, joint, and ligament cells so that next time you work out, your body can handle it better and be stronger. Without inflammation you would never be able to recover from a workout, you would never be able to heal from an injury, you would never be able to recover from sickness, and any exposure to even the mildest irritant would become life-threatening. A healthy inflammatory response is essential to kick-start the healing process so that our bodies could resolve any and all of those issues quickly.

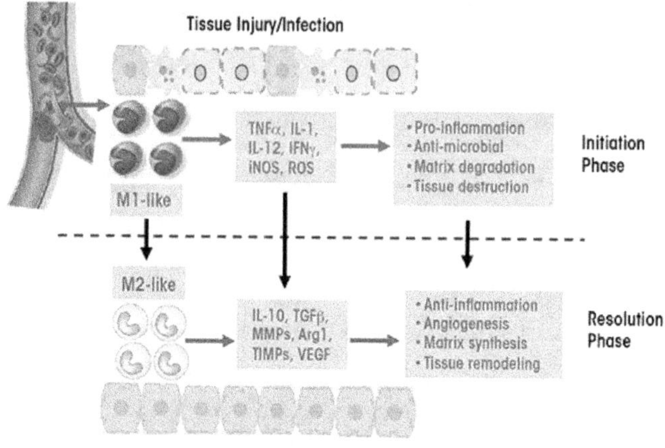

As demonstrated in the image above, one of the mechanisms for how inflammation heals damaged cells is by sending very specific inflammatory markers which destroy the damaged portion of the cell. This happens during the initiation phase. However, for our cells to actually remodel and replace the damaged portion with a new and functional one, it is vital that the cells are in an anti-inflammatory environment. If we remain in the inflammatory state for too long, what will happen is that the same inflammatory markers that destroy the damaged portion of the cell, begin to destroy healthy cells too. And when that goes on for a long time, the body is unable to go through the resolution phase (which is the healing phase), resulting in severe, long term cellular damage.

Another role Inflammation plays in our body is that it serves as a messenger to the brain, notifying it when there is something wrong or damaged in the body so that the brain can take the necessary steps to resolve it. A prime example of this is a fire alarm. When there is a fire in a building, the fire alarm detects the smoke and starts making a loud noise, so that the residents of the building can take the appropriate measure to get out of the building and call the fire department. When a fire alarm is working properly, it can save many lives.

It's the same thing with inflammation, when we have an injured body part, like a strained ankle for example, our immune system triggers the inflammatory process in that area. So what happens to that ankle? It begins to swell up and turn red, which is due to the increased blood flow to that area. The blood then supplies extra oxygen and nutrients to the injured ankle so that the tissues can have the building blocks they need to heal properly from the strain.

Additionally, in a healthy inflammatory response, your ankle should swell up when it is strained. The body sends more blood to that area, then the blood takes the waste products that are produced from the damaged and injured tissues and carries them away to be excreted by the body, thus clearing the way for the healthy tissues to replace the damaged ones. All of this is what happens inside the body when you have a healthy inflammatory response. You can think of it as the clearing out the debris then replacing it with new, healthy, and functional tissue.

This is all good, but if you ask anyone what is their least favorite part of straining an ankle is, they will tell you, "the pain!" Which just happens to be another hallmark symptom of inflammation. This is due to the inflammatory markers increasing pain sensitivity in that area so that you don't continue running on it or overusing it when it is in it is in its vulnerable, damaged state. Could you imagine if you strained your ankle or broke a bone and didn't feel any pain? You would continue to walk on it and use it and you would further damage the strained ankle causing it to take longer to heal.

Pain is one of the body's most effective methods of telling you that there is something wrong in the body. I know the idea of straining an ankle and ignoring the pain and continuing to use it sounds kind of ridiculous, but as you will see in this book, many of us do that with our own vital organs. We unknowingly assault it with the poor lifestyle choices every single day, not allowing our body to have the opportunity to heal and recover from that.

The problem, however, is that the inflammation involved in many health problems such as cardiovascular disease, cancer, diabetes II, allergies, depression, ADHD, Alzheimer's, **is below the threshold of perception of pain.** Meaning, you could have major problems in your heart, or liver, or brain and not feel any pain at all. And there are many people who live their whole lives thinking, "If I don't have pain, then I must be fine, right?" Sadly, that couldn't be any further from the truth.

In the example of the fire alarm, if the fire alarm is ringing and beeping all the time, then that is due to one of two problems. Either there is a fire in your house and the alarm has been ringing for so long that you become desensitized to the noise and begin to ignore it, the outcome of which is fatal. Or the fire alarm is hypersensitive and beeps at any potential stimuli. We have all experienced this at one point, where the fire alarm in our apartment is so sensitive that even boiling water will cause it to go off. The concerning thing about both of these situations is that if there were to be a real fire, you won't even know it, because you would just assume that it is just another "false alarm". Both of these scenarios closely resemble the problems that can happen in our bodies with chronic inflammation.

As you can see, a healthy inflammatory response serves a vital role in the body and is a part of a healthy healing response, as long as it is **acute** (lasts for a short period of time) and is **localized** (only in the area that is damaged/irritated). When inflammation persists longer than it needs to and becomes **chronic** (lasting for a long period of time) and becomes **systemic** (affecting multiple structures/organs and tissues), then it results in more harm than healing.

Remember, inflammation is a natural immune response to injury, irritants, damaged cells, and/or pathogens. So when any of these things get out of hand and become to be too much for the body to handle, inflammation escalates and gets out of control, resulting in diseases in the body. Chronic inflammation is an indication that things have gotten far too out of control in the body.

So what is it that would cause our body to be in a persistent state of inflammation? There are two primary factors that if not addressed, will cause our body's healthy inflammatory response to go haywire and over time tax and degenerate our cellular and organ function, leading to disease and illness. In these next few chapters, we will be going in-depth about what some of the most popular contributors of chronic inflammation are, how they are destroying your body, and what you can do about it to jumpstart your body's natural healing response.

It is with the best intentions by which we are constantly told to make drastic lifestyle changes in order to healthy, but the good news is that for most people, just as these conditions have developed progressively over time, they can also be progressively reversed, over time. The smallest of actions, done consistently, can have a profound effect on our health. We get to choose if it will be a positive effect or a negative one. To do that we must first identify what all these life-threatening conditions have in common and begin to remove the things that have harmed us and continue to harm us and replace them with things that allow our bodies to heal.

With that being said, one of the most vital and overlooked aspects of developing a healthy inflammatory response, one that rejuvenates damaged cells, one that helps you fight disease and illness, one that helps you recover faster, and feel great, is the **digestive system.** It is arguably one of the most critical systems for whether your inflammatory response will heal or hurt you. Our digestive system is the gatekeeper between the outside world and our cells, tissues, and organs.

When we irritate, damage, and inflame our digestive system, we compromise our ability to absorb vital nutrients, vitamins, minerals, amino acids, and antioxidants. This in return, means, that even when we are eating healthy, our body isn't able to fully utilize the nutritious foods that we are eating. So it is of the utmost importance to make sure that we have a healthy digestive system so that we can have a strong foundation for a healthy life.

THE BODY'S GATEKEEPER
WHERE IT ALL BEGINS

So you are probably wondering, "How does chronic inflammation cause Alzheimer's disease, depression, heart disease, ADHD, obesity, fibromyalgia, etc.?" Well, that is a very good question and to answer that, we must first look at the gut. Hippocrates, who is recognized as the father of medicine, said it best when he said, "all disease begins in the gut.". On an intuitive level, most of us realize that what we put into our bodies will either heal us or hurt us. This is not a new concept by any means. As a matter of fact, most of us can probably even recall our mother insisting on us finishing our broccoli before leaving the dinner time. And even though back then, we thought it was some kind of cruel punishment, as we get older, we begin to realized that she insisted on finishing our vegetables so that we can have the building blocks to grow into healthy adults.

But what most people don't know is that 70% of our immune system is found in our digestive tract. And this is for good reason, since most contaminates, bacteria, pathogens, and invaders will enter the body through the mouth. If our digestive tract was not fully armed with a hefty army of our immune system, we would be in serious risk every time we ate or drank something. As you can recall, inflammation is an immune response, and since 70% of our immune system is found in our digestive tract, you can bet on the fact that our digestive tract plays a direct role in chronic inflammation.

Up to this point, most doctors didn't exactly know the degree our digestive system played in our inflammatory response. It wasn't until the recent discovery of **Leaky gut syndrome** that the matter came to light. **Leaky gut syndrome** is a fairly recent discovery, most doctors didn't know about it, and those who did, didn't recognize it as a real medical condition. Even at the time, this book was written, some doctors completely dismiss it as a genuine health condition. There has been a growing number of scientific evidence emerging that prove that not only does leaky gut syndrome exists, but that it is actually contributed to myriads of health issues, ones that are more common than you think. And because its discovery is so recent, many of the associated symptoms have been wrongly misdiagnosed and thus mistreated. Symptoms such as depression, skin rash, fatigue, achy muscles, poor sleep, brain fog, digestive issues, and the list goes on. Do any of these sound familiar to you?

So what is leaky gut syndrome and how exactly is it tied to chronic inflammation? To answer this we first have to review some basic anatomy. And I promise I will keep this fun and simple. You can think of the lining of your gut as a gatekeeper, letting in what is good, and preventing what is bad from entering into the body. This is the first line of defense against any potential invaders and is known as **gut permeability.** It regulates the passage of substances and nutrients into and out of the bloodstream. Very simply, gut permeability plays a vital role in our ability to absorb that which is good and give it to the blood, and preventing the bad stuff from entering into our bloodstream.

When you have a healthy gut, the lining of your digestive tract should have small pores that are just big enough to allow the healthy nutrients that you eat to be absorbed into the bloodstream, so that your body can use it properly for energy, healing, and recovery. However, these pores should not be big enough to let in toxins, bacteria, irritants, and pathogens into the bloodstream. Gut permeability is essential for the absorption of nutrients and water while simultaneously protecting the body from pathogens and other harmful invaders.

What happens with leaky gut syndrome, is that the lining of the gut becomes so inflamed that over time the inflammation damages the gut lining, resulting in those small pores losing their ability to stay small, and thus toxins, irritants, and pathogens gain access into the bloodstream. In this situation, the "gatekeeper" is no longer effectively doing its job. With leaky gut syndrome, the gut permeability becomes damaged and that opens up the door for any potential invaders.

But thankfully, our body has implemented a backup plan just in case our gut lining gets damaged. That's where the immune system comes in. Once any of those pathogens enter into the bloodstream, our immune system recognizes that those invaders don't belong there and begins to send the appropriate inflammatory markers and white blood cells to eliminate them. Under normal circumstances, this is a great back up plan for the rare instances where the gut lining gets damaged. But leaky gut syndrome is not a normal circumstance, because with that syndrome our intestinal lining gets so damaged that your immune system is fighting this battle every time we eat. So instead of that immune response being a back up plan, it becomes the primary one.

To make matters worse, leaky gut syndrome is typically caused by specific foods. Meaning every time we eat the wrong foods, we are further damaging our gut lining and consequently, promoting inflammation throughout our digestive tract. Since toxins, pathogens, and irritants now have direct access into our bloodstream they are more likely to enter into the bloodstream and travel throughout the body. The immune system has to work overtime to ensure that those invaders don't get us sick. When we continually eat the wrong foods, ones that irritate and damage the gut lining, we are unknowing promoting chronic inflammation, taxing the immune system, the organs, and the body, leading to dysfunction and degeneration. In severe cases, the immune system becomes so hypersensitive (on extreme alert mode) to any potential threat that it can even begin attacking your own tissues, this is known as an auto-immune response.

The good news is that our bodies are amazingly capable of recovery. With the right steps and information, leaky gut syndrome is not only preventable but in many cases can even be **reversed**. Simply by identifying and treating leaky gut syndrome, I have seen many of my patients overcome conditions such as migraines, chronic fatigue, obesity, gain mental clarity, improved focus, and mood, relief from joint pain, reduced bloating, enhanced athletic recovery, and clearer skin just to name a few.

Everything in this book is presented in such a way as to give you the knowledge, tools, and guidelines to prevent and/or recover from chronic inflammation, thus allowing your body to heal and be healthy. To restore your body's normal healthy inflammatory response. One that works with your body to heal and protect it, not hurt it.

At this point a common question that you may be asking yourself is, "how do I know if I have leaky gut syndrome?" According to Dr. Leo Galland, director of the Foundation for Integrated Medicine, any of the following symptoms may be signs of leaky gut syndrome:

- o   Long-term diarrhea or constipation
- o   Getting sick frequently (weakened immune system)
- o   Brain fog or unprovoked headaches
- o   Excessive fatigue
- o   Bloating
- o   Excess gas
- o   Strong sugar and/or carb cravings
- o   General muscle achiness
- o   Mild/moderate depression

***Disclaimer**- Now, of course, I should mention that if you have any of these symptoms, you should go see your primary health care provider to have them professionally assessed, diagnosed, and treated. Your primary healthcare provider can rule out any serious life-threatening conditions and prescribe you the appropriate treatment if/when necessary. Since some of these signs and symptoms can be due to a wide spectrum of health reasons, from something as mild as eating a bad meal to more serious health conditions, it is important to leave the diagnosing to your health care provider. This book cannot diagnose, treat, or cure anything but is rather a tool to help you regain your health once your health care provider has cleared you and has approved of you moving forward with the material in this book.

Assuming you have been cleared by your health care provider, my rule of thumb is that if you have checked **two or more** of these symptoms, then chances are you may have leaky gut syndrome. Of course, this is a good general guideline but it is by no means definitive. If you did check two or more of these symptoms, don't panic, I want to remind you that with the right steps, leaky gut is totally reversible.

There is no better way to treat Leaky gut syndrome than by eliminating the very thing that causes it. So what causes Leaky Gut Syndrome?   Let's dive right into it.

THE NOTORIOUS GLUTEN
WHAT IS IT? WHY IS IT SO CONTROVERSIAL?

When whole wheat products were released into the food market, it took over the health industry by storm. We had major doctors, medical associations, and athletes endorsing the health benefits of whole wheat products. Whole wheat has more fiber, it isn't bleached like white flour is, and it even has more of the B vitamins. It was very common for my patients to say, "Hey doc, I have started eating healthy, I have now switched from white bread to whole wheat bread, and I even started cooking with whole grain pasta." Theoretically, whole wheat products are the healthier alternative to the foods made from bleached white flour.

It is true, I would rather have any of my patients consuming whole wheat bread or pasta, over the highly processed/bleached white bread or white pasta, since they will be consuming more fiber, vitamins, and minerals. However, this has given people a false sense of health and healing. Even to this day, most of us think we are taking the healthy option when we order our favorite meal with the whole wheat bread, but as you are about to find out, this is one of the most misleading health movements to date, and it is all due to a single protein molecule called "gluten".

Gluten is a protein found predominantly in wheat and other grains. It is what allows the wheat products to stick together, having a "glue" like property, and thus it has earned the name "gluten". Gluten has been part of the human diet since we began the harvesting of grains and using them to make our foods, and besides the fiber found in the wheat, gluten largely contributes to our sense of fullness. We have been consuming wheat and other gluten-containing grains since the agricultural era with relatively no problems at all.

So why is it that all of a sudden, we keep hearing this fuss over gluten? And why does it seem that suddenly, so many people have developed gluten sensitivity? Well, to answer that, we need to realize that historically speaking, the gluten that was naturally found in wheat rarely affected people back then because it was a natural component of the wheat and we had naturally and gradually developed the enzymes necessary to consume and digest gluten with virtually no ill effects. Our bodies were adapted to the gluten and could break it down with ease, thus subsequently it did not pose as a threat at all.

It wasn't until the 1970's, when Norman Borlaug, in his honorable cause to end world hunger, had aggressively modified the genetic components of the wheat grain to be more resistant to insects, extreme weather conditions, and to yield a greater harvest. Theoretically, this would allow for greater yields of wheat and allow more people to consume wheat and wheat-derived products. On pen and paper, this was a great idea that could help feed hundreds of thousands of people all around the world.

Norman Borlaug did receive the noble peace prize for his positive contribution to providing more people with food, and rightfully so. But little did they know at that time, how much of an impact this would have on our overall health.

The wheat we consume now virtually bears no resemblances to the wheat consumed prior to its modification in the 1970s. With this fairly recent and aggressive genetic modification of the wheat grain, not only has the gluten content increased, but it's also a form of gluten that our bodies did not have time to adapt to and thus we were unable to develop the proper enzymatic processes to handle and digest this "super gluten". This super gluten is one of the only protein our body does not know how to digest. And because of that, we are starting to see a staggering rise in gluten related diseases such as leaky gut syndrome, celiac's, and chronic inflammation. According to current statistics, 1 in 100 people will be diagnosed with celiac disease in the United States. However, it is now estimated that about one-third of all Americans have some degree of gluten sensitivity, which is way higher than the current statistics for celiac disease.

The consumption of gluten directly triggers an inflammatory immune response in our body, since our body no longer recognizes it as the gluten that it once was. It has become so foreign that our bodies see it as a potential threat, and because we can't digest it, it irritates the lining of our digestive tract, leading to leaky gut syndrome. It certainly doesn't help that gluten can be very rough on the intestinal tract and its presence is a constant irritation on the gut lining, damaging it more and more over time, thus further promoting an inflammatory response. As mentioned in the last chapter, the constant consumption of this irritating protein on our digestive tract damages the gut lining and is the single largest contributor to leaky gut syndrome.

The diagram on the next page shows some of the most common symptoms triggered by gluten consumption. As you can see on the bottom left of the diagram, there is still a group of people that may have potentially "silent" symptoms even with the most severe form of gluten sensitivity (celiac disease). These are the very unlucky people because they are lead to believe that as long as they feel fine and have no symptoms at this time, then they are healthy, meanwhile, their body is going through a cascade of inflammatory and immune responses that over time really tax the organ systems in the body. These are the category of people that may seemingly all of a sudden develop an auto-immune disease, Alzheimer's, depression, thyroid issues, etc. What I always strive to achieve in my profession is to not only to treat those who are suffering but to also prevent these issues from developing in the first place.

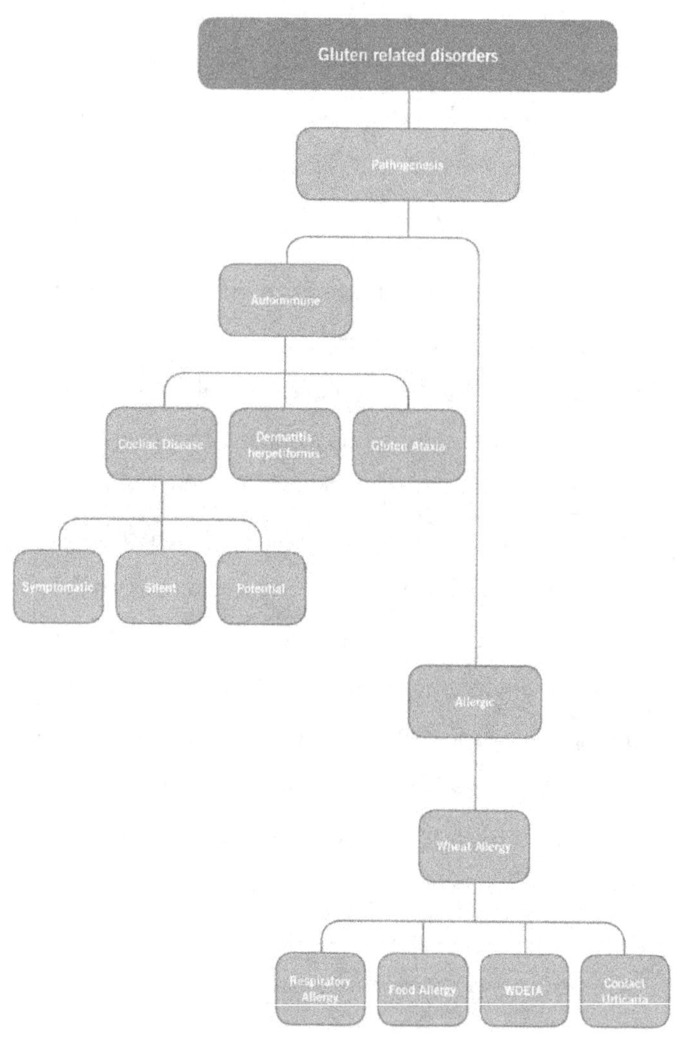

In the traditional American diet, it seems like gluten is virtually unavoidable. Think of some of your favorite foods, pizza, hamburgers, pasta, doughnuts, cake, etc. The flour for the pizza dough, the hamburger buns, and the cake mix all contain a large amount of gluten. For many of us, every time we consume any of these gluten contain foods, we are inflaming our digestive tract, triggering our immune response, and slowly damaging our bodies.

At this stage, you may be wondering, "how is it that gluten can cause diseases in other organs and not the digestive system, as the thyroid, brain, and mood?"

This is where things get really messy with gluten sensitivity, what we see with people who are gluten sensitive is that every time they eat this super gluten protein, they trigger an immune response because their body sees it as a potential invader, thus the body labels it as a threat. And what ends up happening over time is that the immune system becomes hypersensitive to the gluten and attacks anything that closely resembles the gluten protein. When this happens our body's immune system, the very immune system that's supposed to protect us from foreign invaders, pathogens, bacteria, sickness, and from infection; actually ends up attacking our own cells in because they resemble gluten in their structural form. At this stage, gluten sensitivity has become a full-blown autoimmune disease.

Since each person is different and the auto-immune response can have more obvious effects on different organs. Depending on one's unique biological makeup, the immune system can attack brain cells, while for a different person it can attack their thyroid cells, others develop skin issues or may notice the negative effects on their joints. And so even though it may seem that every single one of these issues are not really related, what you may have already began to notice is that they all have the same common cause and it is that chronic inflammatory response.

As you can imagine in this situation, when someone progresses to full-blown autoimmune disease every time they eat gluten containing foods, not only does their immune system attack the gluten molecules but as a consequence it attacks the brain tissue, or thyroid tissue, or joint tissues.

The image on page 42 demonstrates how the white blood cell, known as "helper T cells" find the pathogen/irritant and release powerful inflammatory markers known as "cytokines". The release of cytokines informs the immune system that there is a problem in that area and thus it can send other reinforcing white blood cells. The helper T cells then release more inflammatory enzymes that break the cell membrane of the pathogen or irritant. In a healthy body, with a normal inflammatory response, this process is essential for us to fight disease, sickness, bacteria, infections, and irritants. However, when one develops a full-blown auto-immune disease from their gluten sensitivity, we see that these helper T cells begin attacking our own cells, in this image, our own brain cells. So if your auto-immune response is such that your immune system attacks your own brain tissue every time you eat gluten, then you are will be much more suitable to brain fog, mood disorders, depression, anxiety, and over time even Alzheimer's.

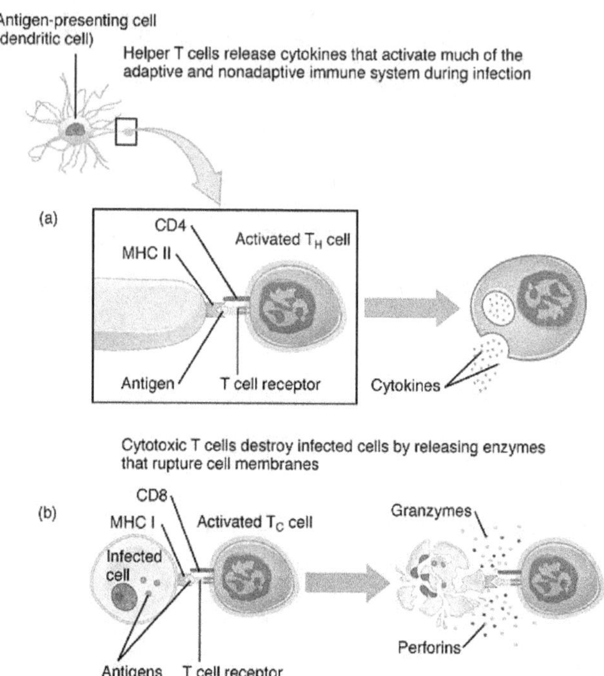

There is even a study published in *Science Journal volume 191*, of a psychiatrist who had a patient with full-blown medication-resistant schizophrenia. He tried nearly every standard treatment for this condition, with no success what so ever. Eventually, he decided to try an unconventional approach and have his patient completely eliminated the gluten from her diet. She began to show improvement in as little as a few days, and within a few weeks, she became a fully functional member of society with no symptoms of schizophrenia whatsoever. Being a man of science, he was utterly shocked by this miraculous transformation. So he instructed her to return to her normal diet and consume her favorite gluten containing foods. Just as he suspected she began to show signs and symptoms of schizophrenia once again. This was all the evidence he needed to be convinced on the detrimental effects gluten has on some people.

I don't want to alarm you, as this is a pretty atypical case. Clearly, his patient had an abnormally severe gluten sensitivity and responded with symptoms that mimicked schizophrenia. But this case study can serve as a testament to the potentially harmful effects of gluten consumption. What is much more clinically common, however, is to see some of my patient's depression significantly decrease and regain their mental clarity. Some of them find that even their ability to handle stress is greatly enhanced. While others find that they are beginning to have a lot more energy. This is an autoimmune response that not only do we want to catch early but prevent from developing altogether.

STRESS HORMONES, CHRONIC INFLAMMATION, AND THE IMMUNE RESPONSE

A secondary effect that can develop from your body being in this constant state of inflammation and hypersensitive immune response, is that your body begins to truly recognize that it is in trouble. All the feedback mechanisms in the body are alerting the brain that there is clearly a problem going on here. If you are gluten sensitive and continue to consume gluten, making your immune system work overtime day in and day out, and continue engaging in all the habits that trigger the inflammatory response, what will typically happen over time is that your brain will signal your adrenal glands to release more stress hormones, adrenaline, cortisol, etc. That is your body's way of telling you, "Hey pay attention to me, there is clearly an issue going on here! Please attend to it immediately!"

That response if left untreated over time will only amplify the negative and degenerative effects of chronic inflammation. Under normal circumstances, our stress response is supposed to serve as a warning sign that we are in imminent, threatening conditions. Our stress response is also commonly known as the "fight or flight" mechanism, to help us either fight the threatening entity or run away from it, which ever will produce the most favorable outcome.

For instance, imagine you were hiking in the woods and all of a sudden you hear a rustling sound in the bushes nearby, you turn around and see a vicious mountain lion and by the looks of it, it hasn't eaten in a long time. Upon recognition, your brain will signal your adrenal glands to pump out adrenaline, cortisol, and other stress hormones to give you a boosted advantage whether you chose to fight it or run away from it. Once that mountain lion disappears, our stress response should lessen and we should be able to return to our normal state once the threat is gone.

However, when your body is in a chronic state of inflammation, when your immune system is constantly fighting this battle against gluten, the brain will recognize these patterns as a health threat and start signaling our stress response to be ramped up. Obviously it will not be as amplified as when you are staring face-to-face with a wild mountain lion, but it gets elevated above normal, and this over time creates a lot of havoc on the body. Ironically enough, when most of us feel stressed, we tend to turn to our favorite comfort foods, foods like pasta, pizza, cake, ice-cream. Most comfort foods will have a large amount of gluten and/or sugar, further triggering this hormonal cascade, even though they will provide you with temporary relief and comfort, over time it can do a number on your body. If only we would turn to our favorite fruit or a greens smoothie when we are feeling stressed, because that is what our bodies so desperately need. The good news, once again, is that all of this is can be reversed, assuming you don't have complicating factors and follow the guidelines and principles in this book, or unless otherwise specified by your personal health care provider.

The image on the next page demonstrates the pathway of our brain signaling our adrenal glands to release stress hormones, which gets released into our bloodstream, thus effecting virtually every cell in the body that gets blood supply.

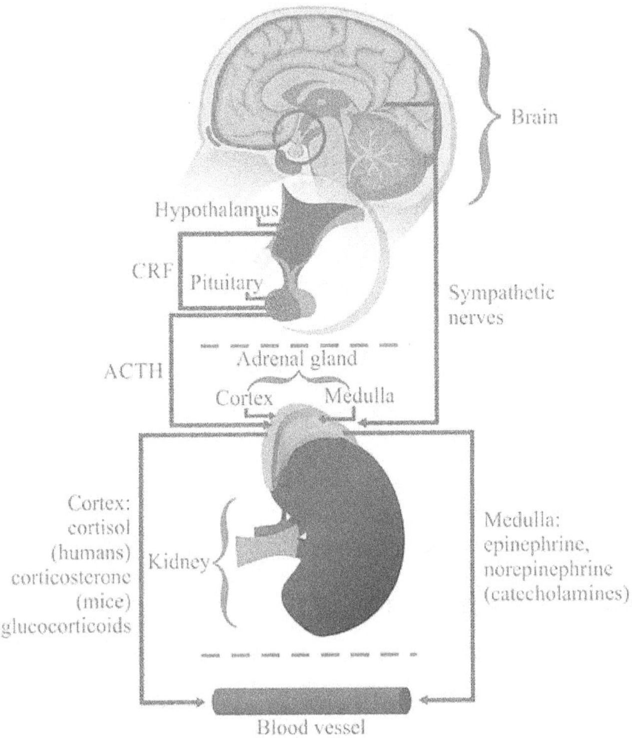

WHY IS GLUTEN SO CONTROVERSIAL?

With all of that being said, why is there so much controversy surrounding gluten? Shouldn't it be obvious by now that it is harmful for our health? Well, One of the biggest reasons why gluten has been so controversial in the health field is due to that fact that people vary in their sensitivity to gluten. Meaning different people react to it in different ways. Some people are extremely sensitive to it, to the point of developing severe mood disorders, skin rashes, and even joint pain whenever they consume something with gluten. While others may just gain weight and have a general sense of brain fog, low energy, indigestion, and think that it is just the way that they are. When in reality these can also be symptoms of a milder form of gluten sensitivity. And of course, there are some people who have no adverse health effects from low to moderate gluten consumption. It is primarily for this reason that gluten has become so controversial. The medical community already recognizes those who are extremely sensitive to gluten, as having celiac disease. Thankfully, there is very little debate as to whether this is a real diagnosable disease or not. But for anyone who is below the threshold of being diagnosed with celiac disease, well, they are typically misdiagnosed or told that it is all in their head. Can you imagine how frustrating that must be?

This wide range of people's reactions to gluten has led to the highly controversial nature of gluten consumption. To make matters worse, there really isn't an accurate way to directly measure the person's degree of gluten sensitivity. Testing for gluten sensitivity is a complex and fairly expensive process. Take a look at the medical flowchart on the next page showing the complexity of diagnosing gluten sensitivity. There are many specific immunoglobulins that need to be tested in the right order before your health care provider can reach a conclusive diagnosis. If you are looking at this flowchart and wondering what language this is written in, you are not alone. Unless you have a lot of time and money, most people will not want to do all this testing. Even if they wanted to, there aren't too many healthcare providers that will offer this level of testing. But do not worry, later in this chapter I will tell you what is a much easier and more affordable way to determine whether you may be getting negative side effects from gluten consumption.

Dr. Mina Botros

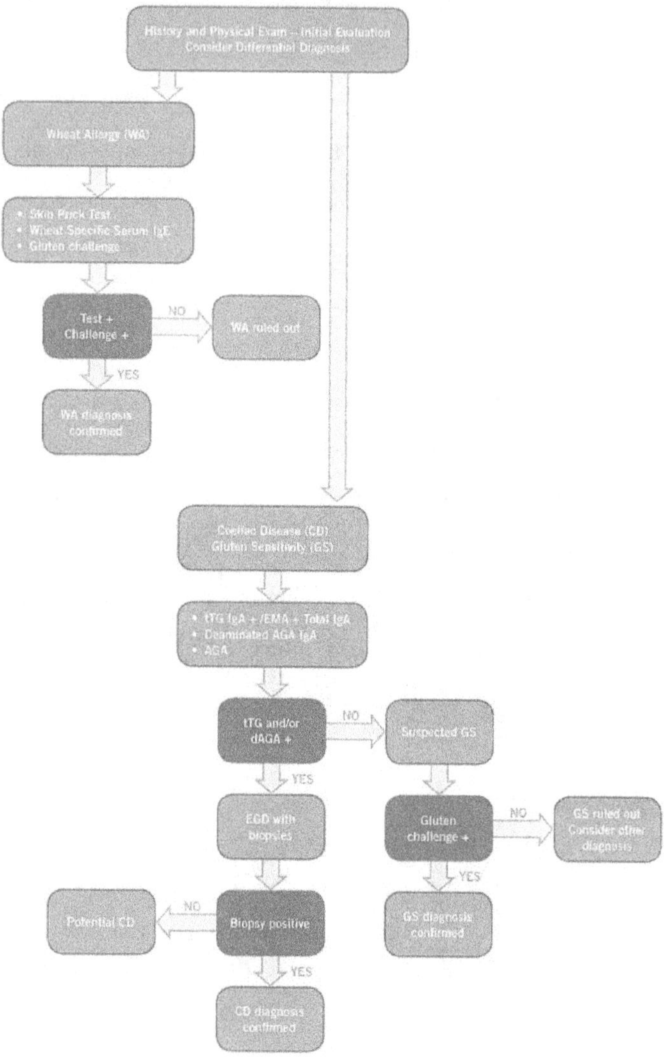

You may be wondering where I stand in this gluten controversy, based on my professional opinion is gluten bad or good? I will give you the most honest and diplomatic answer, in my humble opinion having treated and worked with countless patients,

"It is without a doubt in my mind that everyone who has reduced or eliminated gluten from their diet, has objectively and subjectively felt and became healthier."

- Dr. Mina Botros

All across the board, from my clinical experience and my personal experience, the simple act of reducing the consumption of gluten containing food in my patient's day to day diet, has yielded measurable and noticeable health benefits. Not only is this a concept that I introduce to my patients who want to get out of pain, reduce their risk for chronic disease, and just have an elevated sense of wellbeing. But this is something that I personally noticed in my own health and wellbeing. With some rare exceptions, my gluten consumption is fairly low on a daily basis.

Simply by reducing the amount of gluten I consume, I've noticed that I can think clearer, have more energy, have lost weight and kept it off, and my quality of sleep has improved tremendously. The beautiful thing is that all the things in this book have a compounding effect, meaning that your results can potentially get exponentially better for every lifestyle modification you take towards achieving your true health.

If you really want to test the degree of gluten sensitivity, there are specialty clinics and doctors that have dedicated their whole practice to gluten testing and management. You can typically find them with a quick search online or have your wholistic doctor refer you to a good one. They tend to be rare and highly in demand. Obviously going to a specialty clinic that will test the wide spectrum of specific immune response associate with gluten sensitivity is the gold standard. However, there is a more affordable alternative. It may require a little more effort on your part but it is well worth it. What you can do, is completely eliminate gluten for at least two weeks (you may even have to do it for a month if you are more symptomatic), and see what changes happen. If that seems challenging, you can view it as a fun 30 day challenge, it will allow you to be creative at exploring other food options that are gluten free. When you do this you will notice a pattern that most "gluten free" goods tend to be unprocessed, whole foods found in nature. This by default will allow you to increase your fruits and vegetables, which has nice added health benefits.

This is a challenge I love giving to some of my patients, and I hate to spoil the results that they get but those who stick to it typically report losing an average of 8 pounds, having mental clarity, better digestion, and a sense of well-being. That's not a bad list of improvements from just eliminating gluten. Now I should state that this doesn't happen immediately, for most people, it takes about a week and half to two weeks before they notice the benefits. Let's say you decide to take the 30 day gluten-free challenge, keep a journal, see how much energy you wake up with, pay attention to how you feel, how you think, your overall demeanor throughout the day, your bowel movements, what is your current body weight, and anything else that comes to mind. Monitor these things over the next 30 days and see if you notice any objective and subjective improvements from when you first started.

On the next page, I have added a questionnaire that can help you determine your overall health baseline. You would fill this out at day 1 of eliminating gluten from your diet and then fill it out again at day 30. Then you can compare your results and see which areas improved and which areas stayed the same. You may be pleasantly surprised when you compare your day 30 results with your day 1 answers. That was certainly the case for me and many of my patients. What I like about this is it can be a good gateway into taking control over your health. You get to directly see the role food plays on your body and the kind of results you can achieve in just 30 days.

Systemic Gluten Sensitivity Checklist- circle any of the relevant symptoms on the 0-10 scale, with 10 being very severe symptoms and 0 being not symptomatic at all.

Today's Date: ______________________

1. Headaches   0-1-2-3-4-5-6-7-8-9-10

2. Fatigue   0-1-2-3-4-5-6-7-8-9-10

3. Brain Fog   0-1-2-3-4-5-6-7-8-9-10

4. Depression   0-1-2-3-4-5-6-7-8-9-10

5. Thyroid Dysfunction   0-1-2-3-4-5-6-7-8-9-10

6. Bloating   0-1-2-3-4-5-6-7-8-9-10

7. Stomach Discomfort   0-1-2-3-4-5-6-7-8-9-10

8. Skin Rash/Itchiness   0-1-2-3-4-5-6-7-8-9-10

9. Painful Menses   0-1-2-3-4-5-6-7-8-9-10

10. Achy Muscles/Joints   0-1-2-3-4-5-6-7-8-9-10

***Score:** _____________

*Now add all the numbers that you have circled together and write the sum above in the "Score" section. You can think of this as your current gluten sensitivity score. I have included the exact same test again at the end of the book, so that you can compare your score from before and after you complete the 30 day gluten free challenge.

Systemic Gluten Sensitivity Checklist- circle any of the relevant symptoms on the 0-10 scale, with 10 being very severe symptoms and 0 being not symptomatic at all.

Today's Date: ______________________

1.	Headaches	0-1-2-3-4-5-6-7-8-9-10
2.	Fatigue	0-1-2-3-4-5-6-7-8-9-10
3.	Brain Fog	0-1-2-3-4-5-6-7-8-9-10
4.	Depression	0-1-2-3-4-5-6-7-8-9-10
5.	Thyroid Dysfunction	0-1-2-3-4-5-6-7-8-9-10
6.	Bloating	0-1-2-3-4-5-6-7-8-9-10
7.	Stomach Discomfort	0-1-2-3-4-5-6-7-8-9-10
8.	Skin Rash/Itchiness	0-1-2-3-4-5-6-7-8-9-10
9.	Painful Menses	0-1-2-3-4-5-6-7-8-9-10
10.	Achy Muscles/Joints	0-1-2-3-4-5-6-7-8-9-10

***Score:** ______________

*Now add all the numbers that you have circled together and write the sum above in the "Score" section. You can think of this as your current gluten sensitivity score. I have included the exact same test again at the end of the book, so that you can compare your score from before and after you complete the 30 day gluten free challenge.

THE NOT SO SWEET EFFECTS OF SUGAR

When I was a child, I remember looking forward to getting candy in school for my good behavior. This was a very common practice back then and despite all the current research about the negative effects of sugar, we still reward our kids with sugary treats to this very day. Back then it might not have seemed unharmful, but now there is more data than ever suggesting otherwise.

Most people have a very intimate relationship with sugar, even the expression of "having a sweet tooth" has become a familiar one, most people don't even think twice about it. Desserts and treats have become an iconic part of our culture. We associate positive memories, celebrations and even turn to them as comfort foods, when we feel stressed. However, now we are starting to see that the effects of sugar are in fact, not so sweet.

According to the American Heart Association guideline, the average sugar consumption for an adult in the United States is set around 36 grams! That's not 36 grams per meal, or per snack, but per day! Most of us will exceed that amount just by drinking one can of soda, or a large cup of orange juice. If you compare that to the amount of sugar that the average American adult actually consumes, we are consuming, on average, more than 6 times the recommended amount at any given day.

But, surely the overconsumption of sugar, can't be that bad can it? Well, to answer that question, simply put, sugar consumption has reached epidemic levels. And the worst part is that the sugar epidemic is an epidemic that is hiding in plain sight. It is one that rarely gets any publicity and most people think that sugar is a generally okay for health. It is for those very reasons that it has reached such alarming levels. This is also why it has taken us so long to realize that "sugar" doesn't just apply to sweet things.

Allow me to explain.

CARBOHYDRATE METABOLISM INTO GLUCOSE

When we eat food, our body digests it and breaks it down into smaller units of nutrients and energy so that we can perform our day-to-day tasks, be healthy, and function properly. When we eat a meal that contains carbohydrates and sugars, our body begins the digestive process by breaking down those carbohydrates and sugars into their smallest most usable form of energy, known as glucose. Once your body has broken them down into glucose, your cells can actually begin to use that glucose for cellular functions. You can see it as cellular fuel. So the consumption of carbohydrates is not a bad thing because we do need to consume carbohydrates to be able to have glucose for our body to use for optimal function and health.

As demonstrated in the diagram on the next page, when we consume carbohydrates our body breaks it down into glucose and either uses it for energy or stores it for a later use. Interestingly, our body can actually create glucose from the fats and proteins that we eat. This is really important to note, because it means that if we ever don't get our daily needs of carbohydrates, our body can still supply a steady stream of glucose from either the fat that we ate or from the fat that's stored in our body. Likewise in very extreme cases of starvation if we run out of fat our body can break down the protein in our muscle to convert that to glucose for energy to survive. And as you can see if we eat too much glucose our body naturally begins to store it as fat.

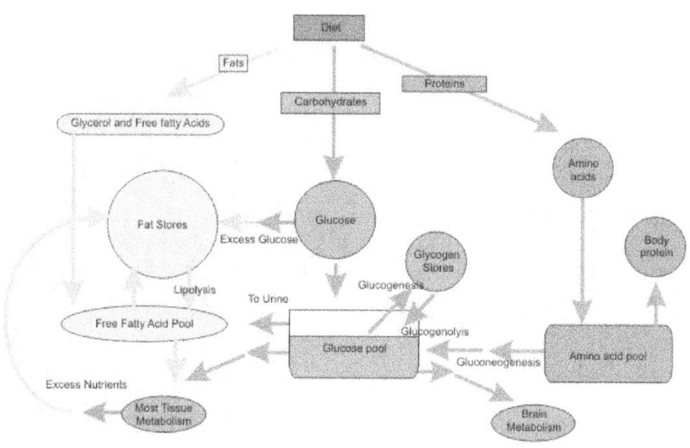

Metabolism Summary

Contrary to popular belief, our body actually doesn't need as much glucose as we had initially thought. Most people can get all their glucose needs simply from eating 100 to 150 g of carbohydrates a day. As a matter of fact, most people can greatly benefit from reducing their carbohydrate consumption to that range. We would have less obesity, less inflammation, less diabetes, more energy, and so many other health benefits.

The problem arises when we consume too many carbohydrates and/or too many sugary products. Why? Well what most people don't know is that table sugar is already broken down into the glucose form, so when you are consuming something with sugar in it, you're already consuming it in its most basic form of energy. This might sound like a good thing and in some cases it is, but for most of us, consuming more than the recommended amounts of sugar per day, can actually lead to many health ailments. These simple sugars are ideal for situation where someone has really exerted their body and they need glucose immediately (like an athlete) or someone who has very low blood sugar and needs to raise it immediately. But for most of us when we are consuming highly sweetened products we are consuming far too much glucose than our body needs and different mechanisms begins to happen in the body as a response to all that sugar consumption that actually ends up hurting us more than helping us.

In order for our body to be healthy it require a steady

stream of energy, in other words it needs a steady stream of glucose. This is measured in blood sugar levels so when we see an individual's the blood sugar are within normal range then we know that their body has a sustained level of glucose in the blood. What we don't want is highs and lows when it comes to our blood sugar levels. Our body prefers them to be stable in order for us to be the healthiest and to be able to function and perform at our best. When we consume highly-processed carbohydrates or sweet products like cake, brownies, and candy, they contain so much sugar that it causes a huge spike of sugar in our blood. Now having elevated blood sugar levels for a long time can actually be quite dangerous and can really damage our cells. I will talk more about how sugar damages our cells later on in this chapter. In the meantime, food manufactures can be very deceiving with the sugars that they put in their foods.

Take a look at the laundry list of sugars that can be hidden in our everyday food. Even the food labeled as "healthy" can have a high amount of those sweeteners.

Common Manufacturing Names for Added Sugar

Dextrose	Sucrose	Maltose	Date sugar
Treacle	Fruit puree	Brown rice syrup	Diastatic malt
Brown sugar	Honey	Fructose	Sorghum
Trehalose	Fruit juice concentrate	Glucose solids	Panocha
Fruit sugar	Beet sugar	Molasses	Turbinado sugar
Evaporated cane juice	Galactose	Raw sugar	Natural sweetener
High-fructose corn syrup	Corn syrup	Demerara sugar	Nutritive sweetener
Invert sugar	Maltodextrin	Malt syrup	Agave nectar

INSULIN

When our body recognizes that our blood sugar (glucose) is too high, the pancreas produces a hormone called insulin which helps clear out the blood from any excess sugar to try to prevent the damage of having elevated blood sugar. In this way our blood sugars can begin to return back to the normal range.

How insulin does that specifically is by taking the glucose from the blood and storing it wherever your body needs it at that particular moment. So if you're an athlete and you worked out hard and your muscles really need glucose to recover from that workout, then once you eat something with sugar, your insulin hormone will send the glucose from the food into your muscles to replenish your muscles natural glucose content. That way next time you workout or play a sport your muscles will have the energy that they need to be strong and have the endurance to perform well. However most of us consume far too much sugar, way more than what we actually need. Thus this raises the amount of glucose in our blood, so our insulin levels begin distributing the excess sugar into our storage cells, which are also known as our fat cells.

As far as your body is concerned having all that extra glucose might come in handy when you are in a situation where you are unable to eat for a long period of time. This mechanism actually allowed us to survive during times of famine and extreme starvation but thankfully that's not a problem that most of us reading this book now face. Most of us are living a very sedentary lifestyle and yet we are consuming more sugar than most professional athletes even need to replenish their muscle glucose levels. Remember according to the American Cardiovascular Association the average American is consuming more than six times recommended levels of sugar.

Just when you think that this is bad enough, sadly, things do get worse. When you consume high sugar and/or highly processed carbohydrates, they cause our body's blood sugar to rise very rapidly and to such high levels, so your pancreas responds by producing insulin, which removes the sugar from our blood stream and stores it as fat, causing our blood sugar levels to drop. And you know what happens when our blood sugar drops after being so high? We feel hungry, agitated, tired, moody, weak, etc. You can see this very clearly with children because their bodies are so effective at this process. You give a child some candy, sweet cereal, a can of soda and all of a sudden they are bouncing off the walls with tons of energy, then followed up shortly with a severe crash. That crashing is due to the insulin removing the sugar from the blood stream. Generally, the greater the rise in blood sugar, the greater the drop. So it is in our best interest to keep our blood sugars at a healthy and stable range, allowing us to have long lasting energy, without the crash, without the hormonal and mood disruptions.

As demonstrated in the flowchart on the next page, what is supposed to be a healthy hormonal cycle to insure our blood glucose levels are stable throughout the day, ends up going haywire when we overwhelm it with consuming too much sugar and/or processed carbohydrates.

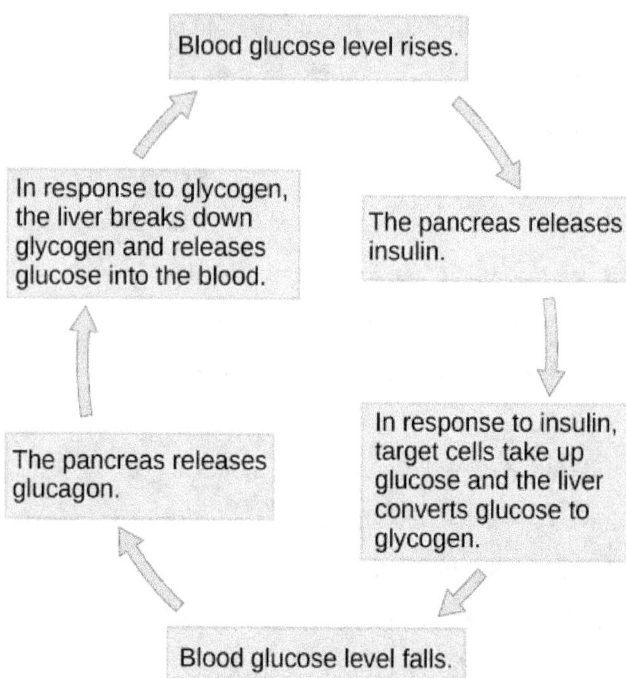

Some people when they learn about the negative effects of sugar get concerned about eating fruits. The good news is that, when you take a look at the carbohydrates found in nature you'll see that most carbohydrates found in nature also contain high amounts of fiber. The fiber found in the carbohydrates found in nature such as in potatoes, tomatoes, blueberries, avocados, apples, etc. Act as a sort of buffer in the digestive process.

So when you consume a piece of fruit with its fiberous skin, not only are you getting the health benefits of fiber but the fiber actually slows down your body's ability to digest that piece of fruit or vegetable. This kind of makes it time released. So even though a piece of fruit may have a high content of sugar, the fiber helps slow down that insulin response and can actually provide you with a steady stream of energy.

Fruit juice on the other hand is a different story. Juice is extracted from a lot of different fruit and it contains no fiber whatsoever and so when you consume it, it is as if you ate three oranges with no fiber. And since it's in liquid form, it's very easy for your body to absorb it thus causing a huge rise in blood glucose levels and a huge insulin spike and even weight gain. Overall, I recommend looking at a cup of fruit juice as if it were a cup of soda. Of course if you had to chose one, the fruit juice is healthier. But overall, if we can reduce our fruit juice consumption, we would be doing more good than harm.

INSULIN RESISTANCE

What happens when we are constantly going through this roller coaster ride of high and low blood glucose and insulin levels? Over a long period of time, we begin to notice a phenomenon known as insulin resistance. What insulin resistance is, is when your body is going through this rollercoaster of producing a ton of insulin to try to regulate and bring down your blood glucose to normal levels. Overtime the receptors on the cells that respond to your insulin hormone become weakened, damaged, and desensitized to the insulin hormone. What this means is that your pancreas will have to release even more insulin to get the message across.

Think of it this way, let's say you've never drank any coffee before, then you take your first couple of sips and immediately you notice the effects that it has on you. You get a sudden surge of energy, feel more focused, even a slight sence of euphoria. After a week of drinking half a cup of coffee, you noticed that you no longer get these effects so you increase the amount of coffee drink to a full cup, and you are happy again. Then after a few more weeks, one cup of coffee is just a part of your routine, you don't get that energy surge that you used to anymore, so you drink a second cup. Just as your body adapts and becomes desensitized to the caffiene, your body can become desensitized to the insulin that you produce. Thus you would have to produce even more insulin than normal, just to lower your blood sugar levels.

This doesn't just happen with caffeine and insulin but with alcohol and drugs too. Overtime the receptors in your body adapt to the stimuli and become desensitized to it. So now every time you're eating carbohydrates your insulin isn't able to effectively do its job so your pancreas has to work overtime to produce even more insulin. Unfortunately, since the insulin is unable to do its job properly, your blood sugar levels get high and stay high. That also means that the cells that actually do need glucose are unable to receive the amount that they need, because the insulin isn't effective at taking the glucose in your blood to give it to the cells that need it. As you can see in the image on the next page, with insulin resistance, the cell's surface is damaged and the insulin is unable to bind to it properly, so the glucose accumulates around the cell, further damaging it. You can also see in that image, that the blood glucose is going to remain high, while the the glucose in the cells remain low. In this case, the person is literally on a biological and cellular level, starving even though they may be physically obese.

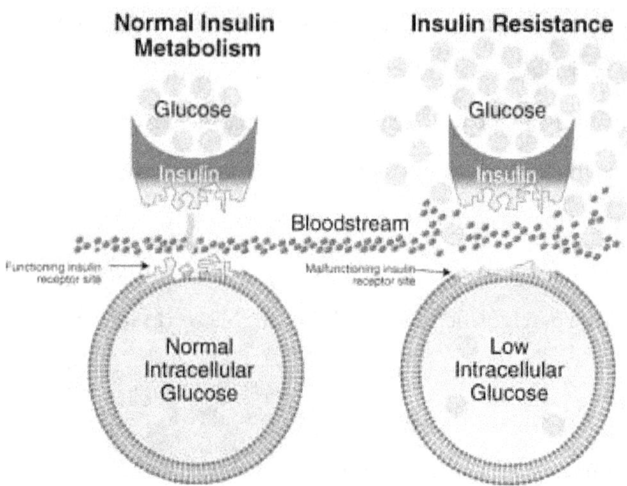

Since the cells are deprived of this essential nutrient (glucose), they begin to collectively signals to the brain that they are not getting the proper energy/fuel (glucose) that they need to function. So the brain releases more hunger hormones so that you can consume more food, in hopes that you will have more food to break down into more glucose, so that the cells may be feed properly. Of course if this continues on for long enough, the person develops **type 2 diabetes**. At the time of this book being writen, diabetes effects 1 out of 10 americans, and 90% of those diagnosed with diabetes have type 2 diabetes, which is the preventable and curable form.

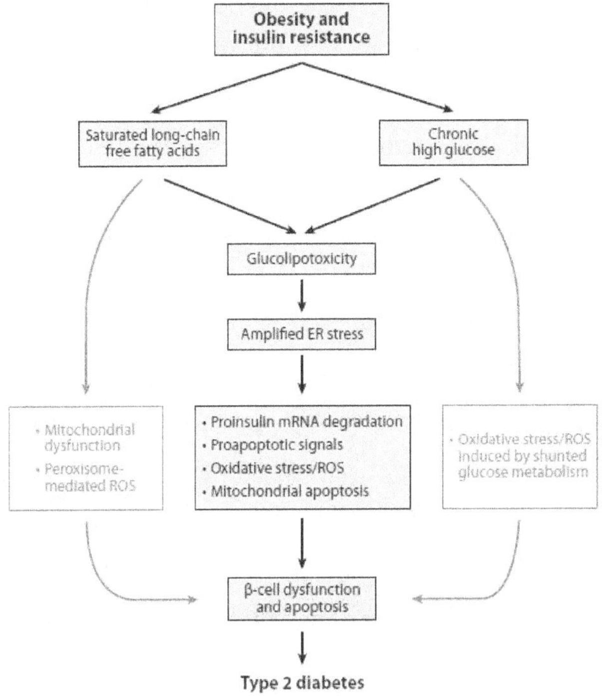

This sudden rise and drop of blood sugar and your body trying to adapt to it by producing more and more insulin to try to stabilize your blood sugar levels can be very taxing on the body. An example I like to give to my patients is imagine if you had a luxury car and poured orange juice into the engine instead of oil, what would happen? All the fine moving pieces of the engine will stick together and instead of having a well-oiled machine, you'll have a damaged and poor running engine. No one in their right mind would do that to their luxury car, or any car for that matter, but we do that with our body all the time. Every time we consume highly processed and inflammatory carbohydrates and sugars and our blood sugar levels rise to unnaturally high levels, we are preventing our body from being a "smooth well-oiled healthy machine".

Over time the processed carbohydrates and sugars damage our cells and tissues, preventing them from functioning properly, which further promotes the inflammatory process. This is your body's way of trying to undo the damage. And as long as we continue to consume excess sugar, soda, fruit juice (which has a lot of sugar), highly processed carbohydrates; our bodies don't stand a chance of optimal healing. Instead of supplying our cells with revitalizing foods and nutrients, we assault them with highly inflammatory foods. Imagine what that is doing to your digestive system, your cardiovascular system, your nervous system.

HOW SUGAR DAMAGES THE BODY (A.G.E.)

To understand the devastating effects of excess sugar on the body we must first understand the concept of free radicals. A free radical is an atom that is missing an electron, thus making them highly reactive and unstable.

Since free radicals are missing an electron what they do is find an electron and steal it for themselves. Now where do they find these electrons? In our healthy cells. Every time a free radical steals an electron from a healthy cell, that healthy cell becomes damaged. It loses its ability to function properly, it become weaker, its life span shortens, etc. In short, free radicals are bad, very bad.

The image below shows an atom that is missing an electron, thus creating a free radical.

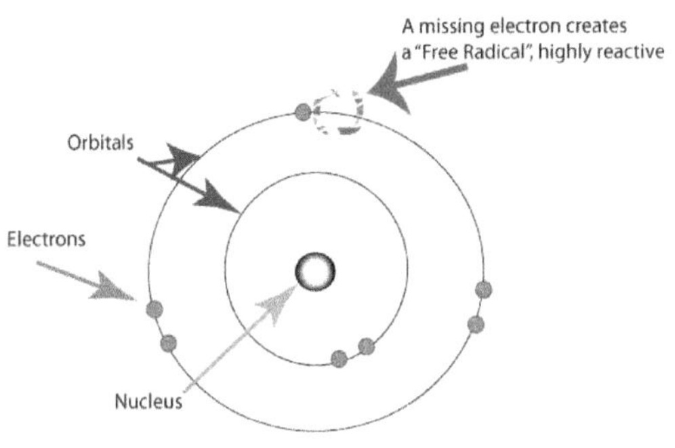

You are probably wondering, how this relates to sugar consumption. Well, every time we eat more sugar than we need, the extra sugar molecule (glucose) binds with any protein and/or fat that's in our blood stream. It is important to note that at any given moment our blood stream contains proteins and fats, as to continuously supply our body with nutrients. Whenever those proteins and fats get exposed to the glucose, however, they react together become "glycated", which in return produces something called "Advanced Glycation End Products", these are also known as A.G.E. among the scientific community. And to answer your next question, yes they do significantly contribute to accelerating the aging processes in the body, but I will talk more about that later in this chapter.

These guys are major trouble, do you remember those "free radicals" we had talked about earlier in this chapter? Advanced Glycation End Products create a lot of free radicals in the body, which in return damages our healthy cells, and makes them much more susceptible to disease, dysfunction, and early cellular death. And as we already know, whenever there is cellular damage or irritation, the body responds by promoting more inflammation to try to heal those damaged cells.

Since most of us are continuously over consuming sugar, and we are constantly producing those A.G.E. products, this is over time damaging our cells. These damaged cells promote the inflammatory response, but since we are constantly damaging our cells through sugar consumption, we shift from promoting a healthy and natural inflammatory response to being in a state of chronic inflammation. And as you already know, over time, if enough cells become damaged and dysfunctional, then you get sick.

Unfortunately, no cell is immune to this process, meaning that every cell can be damaged by the production of advanced glycation end products and free radical. There are, however, some cells that tend to be more sensitive to these advanced glycation end products and are thus more likely to cause problems and manifest in symptoms sooner.

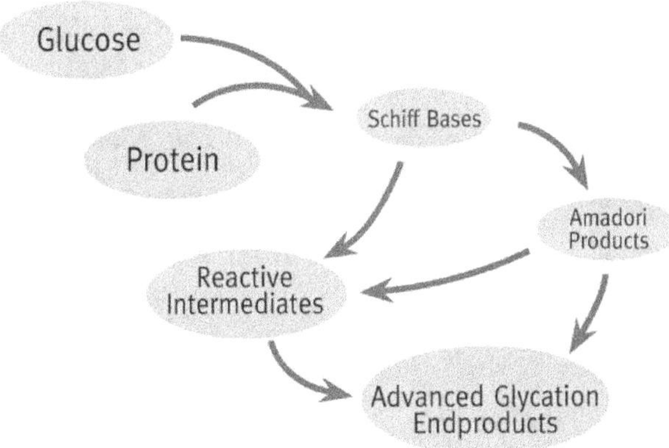

TYPE 2 DIABETES AND ALZHEIMER'S DISEASE

Type 2 diabetes is really the disease of insulin resistance, and with insulin resistance comes a host of many health risks. Even if your insulin resistance isn't severe enough to be diagnosed as Type 2 diabetes, it is very important to be aware of what high sugar and processed carbohydrate intake does to the body via promoting a chronic inflammatory response throughout all the systems in the body.

The unfortunate reality is that type 2 diabetes is completely preventable. And it wasn't too long ago when it used to be called "adult onset diabetes", because it was a disease that developed during adulthood from long term consumption of a lot of carbohydrates and sugars. However due to the fact that more and more kids are being diagnosed with this, its name has changed to "type 2 diabetes". Now I should clarify that type 1 diabetes is something that a person is born with and thus it needs to be constantly managed by a doctor and it is not reversable like type 2 diabetes is.

Remember inflammation is your body's way of healing your damaged cells and when you have insulin resistance and your cells' insulin receptors are worn and damaged and thus are unable to bind with the insulin hormone; it's going to promote inflammation and every time you consume excess sugar and/or excess processed carbohydrates you are directly feeding your chronic inflammation.

Not only do we see that type 2 diabetes increases your risk of nerve damage, excess weight gain, heart disease, and stroke; those with diabetes are nearly twice as likely to develop Alzheimer's disease. As a matter of fact some doctors are now beginning to call Alzheimer's type 3 diabetes because of the strong relationship between insulin resistance and the significant role type 2 diabetes plays on the development of Alzheimer's disease.

Chronic inflammation could be damaging our brain and we could be completely oblivious to it till it is too late. Interestingly, the brain itself actually has no pain receptors. So while our ankle hurts when we sprain it, or we get stomach aches when we eat something that doesn't agree with us, our brain wouldn't have that. When it is inflamed, we begin to get brain dysfunction.

SUGAR AND THE BRAIN

As stated earlier, our body and brain requires glucose to function properly, but the amount that we need is actually a lot less than we are lead to believe. So the question that arises is, what does too much sugar/carbohydrate consumption do to the brain?

While most people are aware of the negative effects of sugar on their heart and other organs, they have far less knowledge of how it affects the brain. As a result, many of us go on with our lives attributing the negative effects of sugar to another cause. Thus may people end up going to doctors who treat their symptoms, often not addressing the root cause of what is going on. So with that being said, let's go deep into how excess sugar and/or carbohydrates can negatively impact brain health and function.

We do need carbohydrates in order to produce certain neurotransmitters. Neurotransmitters are the brain's chemical signals that are in charge of how you feel, how you think, your motivation levels, pain, reward, fear, sleep; pretty much our emotions and behaviors. We see when someone has low blood sugar, for example, they can become confused, irritable, fatigued, that is because those neurotransmitters in the brain don't have the proper fuel to do what they need to do.

Although the brain is dependent on glucose as its main fuel and cannot be without it, too much of sugar source can be a bad thing. Even when someone has completely cut carbohydrates and sugars from their diet, the body will find a way to create the glucose it needs from the proteins that you eat. Most of us here in the United States will be facing major health issues not because of too little sugar consumption, but because we are consuming far more than what we actually need to be healthy.

The effects of sugar on the brain may be the most profound in diabetic patients. This is a condition that impairs the body's ability to process and use the glucose in the blood. With diabetes, the body is not able to produce or respond to the hormone insulin, this leads to abnormal metabolism of carbohydrates and higher levels of glucose in the blood. This leads to increased free radical production and the Advanced Glycation End Products, damaging brain cells, neurons, and many other cells in the body.

More so, the fluctuation of blood sugar levels that occur with diabetes can also damage blood vessels in the brain, which research has also found may lower cognitive function.

The longer you have diabetes, the higher the risk for negative consequence on your brain and mental functions. The increased risk of damage to blood vessels in the body and the delicate blood vessels in the brain over time, reduces the amount of blood, oxygen, and nutrients to arrive to the brain and brain cells. This damage can even affect the brain's white matter, the part of the brain where nerves communicate with one another, slowing down your ability to form new thoughts, think sharply, vividly recall memories, etc. When the neurons in the brain are damaged, you can have cognitive difficulties, which could eventually lead to cognitive impairment or even dementia.

SUGAR ADDICTION

The negative effects of sugar on the brain don't stop there though. It can also impair our self-control, causing increased cravings and addiction. When you have even a little sugar, it stimulates the craving for more. Research suggests that sweet foods, just like salty and fatty foods, can produce addiction-like effects in the human brain, leading to a loss of self-control, overeating, and weight gain.

The addiction occurs as soon as the sugary food lands on your tongue. Your sweet sensing taste buds activate and send signals to the brain, releasing the neurological reward system thus causing that feel-good sugar high. Dopamine is one of the key players in this neurological process, it is a neurochemical that regulates motivation, pleasure, and reinforcement related to certain stimuli, such as food. So for your brain to realized that something is good and it wants more, it will release more dopamine to create a reward system. Thus every time you do this "thing" or eat that food, you will feel great… temporarily. But this system can be hacked, we see this with various addictions such as gambling, various substances, porn, etc.

Interestingly studies have shown that diets with a higher glycemic load stimulate regions of the brain linked with the reward response and trigger more intense feelings of over-all hunger compared to diets with a lower glycemic load. Foods that cause a faster rise in blood glucose are the biggest contributors to addictive eating habits for this very reason.

Various studies carried out on brain activity have shown that even overeating alters the brain's reward system, which then encourages more overeating in the future. This occurs because sugar actually can inhibit the brain's anorexigenic oxytocin system from working effectively. This is the sensory system in the body that prevents us from over eating. It is thanks to this system that we don't eat ourselves to death. This same process is believed to be the basis of the tolerance associated with addiction.

Over time, just like with caffeine, with insulin, and with many other things, we become desensitized and thus need progressively higher amounts to reach and maintain the same level of that rewarding/satisfying feeling. I know I have mentioned a lot of studies in this chapter, but I really think it is important to solidify this point, because for most of us, sugar has slipped under our radar for things that can be negatively impacting our health.

We are seeing that obese individuals have a lower number of those reward dopamine receptors in the brain, than lean people. And since their reward response from food is not as sensitive as it is for lean individuals, it is believed that they compensate by overeating. This has suggested that overeating diminishes the dopamine reward response, encouraging more addiction to low-nutrient foods; foods that are rich in sugar, salt, and fat. The good news is that this doesn't mean that if we are obese we are sentenced to being that way forever. We can still make our receptors sensitive and healthy. Reducing sugar consumption can really help with that.

As previously mentioned, having high blood glucose levels for long periods of time can negatively affect the blood vessels. When the blood vessel is damaged, this can result in vascular complications of diabetes, resulting in issues such as damage to blood vessels in the brain and eyes. This is no trivial matter as diabetes damage to the delicate blood vessels in the eyes is the leading cause of blindness among working age individuals in the United States.

Various studies have shown that long-term diabetes leads to progressive brain damage, resulting in deficits in learning, memory, motor speed, and other cognitive functions. Persistent exposure to high glucose levels leads to decreased mental capacity, and has been linked with a greater degree of brain shrinkage as we age. While learning about this it can be pretty shocking to realize that about 90% of diabetic cases are preventable and can be treated mostly through proper dietary changes. The important thing to realize is that the effect of glucose on brain function can be harsh even in those without diabetes.

THE RELATIONSHIP BETWEEN SUGAR AND DEMENTIA

Perhaps the most condemning evidence lies in the research that shows that foods high in added sugar can lower the production of a very important brain chemical known as **brain-derived neurotrophic factor (BDNF)**. This fancy medical word is actually very important as it has been shown to lower the risk of many mental and neurological diseases. More and more emerging studies are coming out showing that low production of BDNF is associated with symptoms of depression, memory loss, slow reaction time, compromised critical thinking and more.

Those with diabetes and pre-diabetes tend to have lower levels of BDNF. And as the amount sugar consumptions increases the amount of BDNF produced decreases. What this means is the excess consumption of added sugar reduces BDNF, additionally eventually leading to insulin resistance. This over time can lead to type 2 diabetes, metabolic syndrome, and a host of other health complications.

We are starting to realize that low BDNF levels are more directly linked to depression than serotonin levels.

Which can indicate that our conventional medication to treat depression may not be treating the root cause of depression. And it may be in our life time that we see that new depression medications will be targeting BDNF instead of serotonin levels. The new research carried out from the University of Bath in the United Kingdom suggests that chronic sugar consumption puts people at higher risk of Alzheimer's disease because excess glucose damages a vital enzyme that is necessary to preventing Alzheimer's disease.

It has already been established that diabetes patients are at an increased risk for developing Alzheimer's. However, the alarming thing is that even non-diabetics who consume excessive amounts of sugar for long periods of time are putting themselves at an increased risk of developing Alzheimer's disease.

While studying brain samples from people with and without Alzheimer's disease, scientists found that in the early stages of Alzheimer's, an enzyme known as macrophage migration inhibitory factor, (MIF) is damaged through a process known as glycation. Glycation is when the glucose molecule bonds with a protein or fat molecule in the blood.

Researchers think that prevention and reduction of MIF activity caused by glycation could slow down the disease's progression. They also found that as Alzheimer's disease gets worse, it is unsurprisingly accompanied by an increase of glycation of the MIF enzymes. It is for this reason that Alzheimer's Disease is now being referred to as Type III Diabetes.

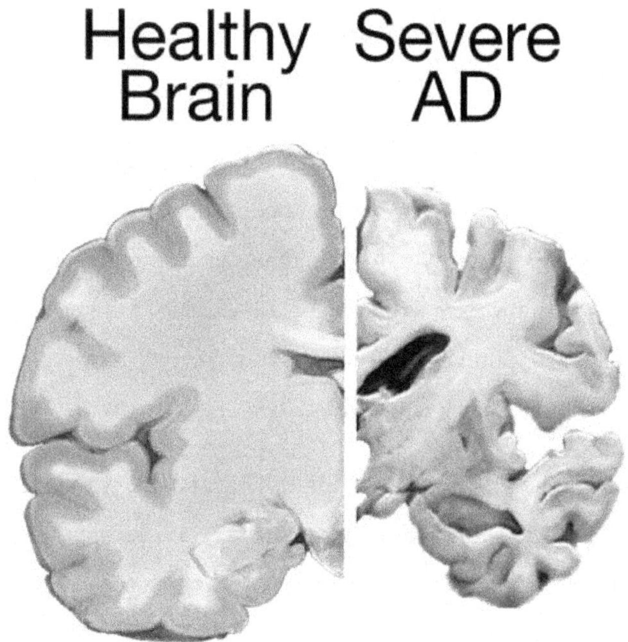

As you can see from the image above of a side-by-side comparison of a healthy brain and a brain with severe Alzheimer's disease. The brain with severe Alzheimer's disease is withered and smaller than a healthy brain.

It may seem like a paradox at first, that our brain actually requires glucose to function properly, but if we eat too much it can be inflammatory to the brain and lead to mental and neurological symptoms. To better understand this paradox, it is essential to first understand the primary needs of brain cells.

As you may already know, neurons require glucose, oxygen, and proper stimulation to function effectively. Whenever we deprive our neurons of glucose, oxygen or even simulation, the outcome is usually not good. That is why solitary confinement of prisoners can be very dangerous, because these prisoners are put in a dark room where there is no visual stimulation at all. This is also why learning a new language, socializing, playing an instrument, traveling, exercising, reading, trying new things, etc. is so wonderful for brain health.

As you can imagine, there is a healthy range in which our glucose levels should be at so that the brain can get the fuel that it needs. Keeping sugar levels stable is crucial to minimizing inflammation in the brain. When the amount of sugar in the blood drops to a level that is too low to sustain normal functioning, this results in hypoglycemia.

The brain will not have the bare minimal fuel it needs to function and do its day to day tasks. On the other hand, when the amount of blood glucose is too high, it results in hyperglycemia and eventually insulin resistance, which opens up a whole new can of worms.

Common Symptoms of Sugar Addiction:

- Eating to relieve fatigue
- Feeling agitated or nervous
- Increased energy after meals
- Cravings for sweets between meals
- Becoming light headed if meals are missed

Common Symptoms of Insulin Resistance:

- General fatigue
- Difficulty losing weight
- Fatigue after eating meals
- Constant hunger
- Cravings for sweets that are not relieved after eating them

So how do these lead to inflammation? When the amount of sugar in the blood rises to a level that's too high, or when blood sugar levels are continuously raising and dropping, this triggers microglia, a primary immune system cell in the central nervous system and brain.

The activation of microglia directly leads to inflammatory responses in the brain, nerves, and spinal cord. This is known as neuroinflammation. When this occurs for a long period of time and becomes chronic, it can cause damage to the brain's tissue.

Sugar initially is excitatory for the brain. Most of us can recall a time when we eat our favorite ice cream or candy bar and felt our energy levels and mood rise. Usually this is very temporary, after the stimulation wears off, our brain's signals slows down. The ability for the neuron to communicate with each other slows down, setting off that brain fog-like feeling and giving us that mental crash. To tackle this, it is crucial to maintain proper blood sugar levels through a maintainable lifestyle change.

Potential Sugar Alternatives

Your brain does need small amounts of sugar to function normally. This means that you need glucose to keep going, but if you are going to consume sugar, you must consider substituting refined sugar for natural ones. Hence, you can begin to reduce your health risks by consuming fresh fruit. Eating fresh fruits enables you to reap loads of benefits in the form of fiber, antioxidants, and phytochemicals that diminish the rise of blood sugar levels and the sudden spike of insulin in the bloodstream.

Here are some alternatives to sugar you may want to consider if you are looking to reduce your overall sugar consumption;

- **Stevia:** Stevia is a nonnutritive sweetener extracted from the leaves of a shrub in South American. This natural sweetener, which has almost no calories, is used to keep blood sugar levels in check. It can even be used by those who are adhering to the nutritional ketosis diet.

- **Xylitol:** Xylitol is a natural sugar alcohol used as a sugar substitute. This natural sweetener is found in small amounts in many fruits, vegetables, and from the bark of birchwood trees. Xylitol is commonly used as an ingredient in sugar-free diabetes-friendly foods, oral-care products, chewing gums, candies, and mints.

- **Fruit:** Low-sugar, high fiber fruits such as blueberries, blackberries, grapefruit, etc., are an excellent option to satisfy your sugar cravings.

As with any of the suggestions mentioned in the

previous page, these sugar alternatives are not a free pass to consume them excessively. They are a much better alternative to refined sugar, but should still be consumed in moderation.

It is also important to be vigilant with concentrated sweeteners like agave, honey, and maple syrup, since research shows that they also can spike blood sugar levels, and even though they may be marketed as good sugar alternatives, they are not. The same can be said of sucralose, aspartame, and saccharin. These are usually included in a multitude of foods and drinks, such as sugar-free snacks, diet soda, and energy drinks. And it is crucial that you watch out for them if you are looking to keep your blood sugar at healthy levels and avoid the risks of chronic inflammation.

THE BODY'S HEALING RATIO
THE BODY'S PREFERRED METHOD OF HEALING

It may come as a surprise to most people, but healing is a two part process. The first part is to eliminate the things that get in the way of our body's being able to heal. The second part is to provide the body with all the essential building blocks and aids to allow it to heal and recover properly.

In the previous chapters, we unveiled some of the biggest culprits that induce the chronic inflammatory response in the body. Over time, not only do they slow down the body's natural healing process but actually have a degenerative and harmful effect. Up to this point, we went over what foods to reduce/eliminate so that you give your body the best change to heal. That is the first half of the healing ratio. Now I would like to focus on things to increase so that you can give your body the tools it needs to heal properly. It is by approaching health in this way that my patients have been able to get such great results.

The Healing Ratio:

1. You must **"reduce"** anything that harms your body
2. You must **"increase"** the things that promote healing

I understand that this may seem overly simplified, but the reality is that it is often the simple things that we neglect. You have a health ratio, and what you want to focus on is reducing the inflammatory foods, habits, and substances while simultaneously increasing the healthy ones.

It is worth acknowledging the importance of these two steps and the order in which they need to happen for your body to be able to heal properly. The reason most health programs, books, workshops, and transformations fail to deliver lasting results is because we are taught that healing requires us to **"add"** something. We have to "add" this medication, we have to "add" this food, we have to "add" this workout, etc. And that is good, however, it is incomplete. As you probably have recognized, this concept only focuses on the second half of the healing process.

What is often neglected is **"subtracting"** the negative habits, foods, and patterns that interfere with our body's ability to heal. As long as that ratio is incomplete, no matter how hard one tries, the outcome will always be less than what your potential for healing can be. It is like trying to clean your pool by adding more chlorine and antibacterial chemicals, but not removing the dirt, bugs, and dead leaves. Yes, it will be a cleaner pool, but if you removed the dirt and bugs and then added the antibacterial pool chemicals, then you will really have a sparkling pool.

Simply by being aware of this formula and making an effort to reduce/eliminate the amount of sugar, processed foods, gluten, etc. in your diet, you have already done the hardest and most important part of the healing formula. You see, as long as there isn't constant exposure to the inflammatory foods, toxins, and habits, then the body can finally have an opportunity to heal and, overtime, even reverse some of the damage done by chronic inflammation. Just by doing that, you can take comfort in the fact that your body is working the way it was meant to, to recover from the negative effects of chronic inflammation.

Of course, why settle for "good" results, when we can achieve "great" results? We want to super charge our body's ability to heal, to make sure that it has the best advantage to be healthy so we can live the life that we are meant to, one with longevity and high quality. If you decide to discontinue reading this book up to this point of and just do the things mentioned in the previous chapter, you will probably be better off than 85% of the people out there. If this is all that you get from this book, and you follow what has been instructed so far and stay consistent with it, you may be really amazed by the results you can achieve.

However, I wrote this book for people that want to completely transform their lives and health in the shortest amount of time possible and in the easiest ways possible. If you are one of those people then it is important that we don't neglect the second part of the health ratio. We want to jump start and aid the body's natural healing process, so that you can get the best results in the shortest amount of time.

The remainder of the book is going to focus primarily on the simple yet powerful, positive additions to your diet that will give your body the essential building blocks it needs to recover and rejuvenate in record time. Not only will these tips help in that regard but they will also jump start the body's natural healing response allowing you to get relief and recover from some of the issues induced by your body being in a chronic state of inflammation.   It is at this point that I highly recommend going back to the first and second chapter, where you have identified your **"whys"** and your **"whats"**. Because reminding yourself of your goals and why you want achieve them is the secret to creating the momentum and endurance to make all these lifestyle changes.

Many of my patients become different people once they implement the materials outlined in this book. I often like to remind them of how they first walked into the clinic, "how did you look", "how did you feel", "what was bothering you?"   They are often shocked by the transformation they have made, some of them even tear up thinking of how much suffering they were going through back then. Some of my patients genuinely thought that that they were "stuck" that way for the rest of their lives. That being unhealthy, overweight, inflamed, and depressed was the burden they were destined to carry for the rest of their lives.

I have seen some of my patients reduce/eliminate their blood pressure medication, their migraine medication, their over the counter pain medications (all of this was under the supervision and recommendation of their prescribing doctor, of course), some of my patients have lost a signification amount of weight, I've seen patients finally being able to relax and have a good night's sleep, and many more of what I call "mini-miracles".

And as much as I would love to get all the credit for this, it is your body that does all the healing, when we get a cut on our skin, it's the body that recognizes that and heals it. It is the same body that also knows how to get you healthy from the symptoms of chronic inflammation. It is the same body that tells you when you are thirsty, when you are hungry, when you are tired, and when you have to go to the bathroom. These are all signals from your body to tell you to do something. Likewise, when our body gives us negative symptoms, we must listen to what it is trying to tell us. It could be as simple as needing to reduce the inflammation that you have acquired over the years.

I hope that my patients, my family, myself, and you as the reader of this book do not become another statistic when it comes to heart disease, cancer, diabetes, allergies, depression, ADHD, Alzheimer's, etc. I hope that we can change the tide of healthcare. I hope that the remaining content of this book serves you well, that it continues to inspire you to take action in your life and health, so that you too can have your own wonderful transformation story.

With that being said, let us move on to some of the most powerful additions that aid us in this fight against chronic inflammation.

Now, I know the thought of cutting out gluten and sugar completely from your diet can be overwhelming, but take a deep breath in and let it all out. Don't worry, I am here to guide you through this process. One of my favorite quotes when it applies to lifestyle changes is that, **"Reaching your health goals is not a sprint, but a marathon."**

To make true and lasting progress towards our health, the type of progress that will help us reverse leaky gut syndrome, reduce our risk of cancers, obesity, Alzheimer's, diabetes, heart disease, arthritis, depression, ADHD, and all the diseases caused or made worse by chronic inflammation. The type of health where you just exude vitality, one where people ask you, "how did you lose so much weight?" or "how do you have so much energy?" We must first approach any lifestyle change with a "small but consistent" manner. After all, I assume you want to be healthy while still enjoying life, am I right? Sometimes making drastic lifestyle changes can work, but I find that they are difficult to sustain.

One of the primary reasons I have been able to achieve such great success with my patients is because I learned very quickly and very early in practice that drastic lifestyle changes often don't work. At best, with a whole lot of willpower and determination, a person can make some temporary improvements, but it's only a matter of time before they fall back into their old habits. I have seen and experienced this process countless of times both with my patients and with myself; with trying to lose weight, with trying to go to the gym regularly, with trying to quit a bad habit, etc. I call this the "New Year's Resolution Syndrome"! Because every new year, millions of people create New Year's resolution to drastically change their life, yet statistically speaking less than 8% of people actually achieve their goals. I prefer to empower my patients with something that has better odds than a 92% failure rate. The good news is that the 92% of the people who set goals and do not achieve them, are not at fault. It is actually a matter of how our brains are wired.

Once you understand how the brain is wired, then

you can understand how to rewire it. That is what lifestyle change is all about, it is about rewiring our brains in favor of the new, positive habit instead of the old, negative ones. As you go through your journey towards vibrant health, energy, elevated mood and wellbeing, towards having a healthier body that feels great, I would like to introduce you to the first principle of using our brains neurological habits to our advantage instead of being trapped by them. Thus rewiring our brains to develop new, healthy habits that bring us closer to our goals, while simultaneously cutting out the habits that prevent us from living the life we deserve and desire.

"Where Attention goes Energy flows!"

-James Redfield

Principle 1: Focus On What You Can Have, Not What You Can't

Most of us when making any kind of lifestyle change, tend to focus more on the things that we cannot have or the things that we cannot do. Theoretically it makes sense, you have to be cautious so that you don't accidently smoke that cigarette or eat that jug of ice-cream or a whole pizza. Ironically what ends up happening is that because we have focused so intensely on not having that cigarette or pizza, and have unintentionally made it the center of our focus, we actually end up slipping and doing the very thing we were focused on not doing.

Here is a really good example to illustrate this. If I told you, **"Hey, don't think of a pink zebra!"** Did you just think of a pink zebra? Why do you think that is? It's not due to you being rebellious, or disobedient, or having no self-control or will power. Rather it is just the way our brains are wired, we naturally think about the thing that captures our attention. So when I drew your attention to a pink zebra, you thought about it, and imagined it, even if you have never seen a pink zebra before. As ridiculous as this may seem, you would never tell yourself in frustration, "I can't believe I thought of a pink zebra, I must have no willpower what-so-ever!" And just as you wouldn't blame yourself for that, you really can't blame yourself for all those times you tried to quit smoking, cut back on sugar, start exercising, and failed to do so. We are simply not taught how to use our neurological processes for our advantage, so we end up falling victim to them and not understanding why we keep failing at achieving our goals. This can give us the impression that those who have achieved their goals are somehow smarter or stronger than us, but this is not true. We simply aren't fully aware of how to use our brain to its fullest capabilities.

Another very good example of this is "reverse psychology". Have you ever instructed a child not to eat the cookies on the table till after dinner, just to find that by the time you were done preparing for dinner, some of the cookies are gone? Why does reverse psychology work so well (not just in kids by the way)? It is because of the same neurological process described earlier. When you instructed that child to not eat the cookies, what you did is brought their attention to the cookies. So now they are thinking about them, perhaps they are wondering why they have to wait till after dinner to eat them, or perhaps they are thinking that cookies taste best when they are fresh from the oven. In any case, what you have done is planted the cookie in their mind, and because they will be thinking about it, it is so much more difficult to resist. Having to resist it at that stage would require you to use your willpower. Clearly, using willpower alone is a recipe for failure, think of all the New Year's goals that were never achieved. It is because most people think that to achieve a goal, they need to use their willpower. When in reality, our willpower is finite, and when we only rely on it, we eventually run out of willpower. Psychologists have likened willpower to a muscle, we can train ourselves to develop stronger willpower, but like any muscle, if you try to carry more than you can carry, your muscle will fatigue and fail. Willpower is a lot more helpful if we can use it in addition to the principles outlined here.

You see, most lifestyle programs now-a-days are glamorized, exaggerated, over complicated, when in reality they don't need to be. People tend to believe that if they want to make any "real" lifestyle changes that they will need to do something drastic and extreme, but this is rarely the case.

Simply by drawing your attention to the things that you CAN eat, the things you CAN do, the things you CAN have, you increase your ability to cut out a bad habit significantly.

This technique works extremely well with any habits or patterns that you are trying to break, cut, reduce, or eliminate. So I highly recommend that you utilize it when you are trying to reduce/eliminate all the harmful foods that have led to your chronic inflammation. I encourage you to focus on all the vibrant lush vegetables that you can eat, the colorful and delicious fresh fruits, how good it will feel to lose weight, what you are going to do with all of the new energy that you will get, how wonderful it will be to have mental clarity, to do the things that you love, all the savory meals you can prepare without gluten, etc. There are many gluten free recipe books, and articles online. There are many fun recipes that you can create that are excellent for your health, get creative and have fun with it. Get excited about all the things you can have, eat, and do.

It is important to recognize that this last technique is extremely effective in eliminating or reducing a bad habit. It allows you to use your brain's reward system to your advantage, instead of having it working against you. This in return allows you to not have to rely strictly on your own willpower. It is easy to break a positive streak when you begin to think about all the things that you are missing out on. We tend to romanticize how delicious that piece of dessert would be, and all of the creative ways we would eat it. But by simply changing your focus on the abundance of delicious foods, dishes, and benefits you can achieve; you will find that life is a lot easier and change can is more enjoyable this way.

If you are trying to add a new habit however, that is

going to require a different technique, as developing new habits utilize a completely different neurological mechanism in the brain.

Principle 2: Adding a New Habit, Starting is The Hardest Part

When it comes to adding a new habit, getting started is the hardest part. Think of all of the times you told yourself that you will start a new exercise program, or that you will eat broccoli every day, or wake up earlier, drink more water, or perhaps you told yourself that you will start your morning with a prayer or meditation. Now think of all the times you started doing these things enthusiastically, just too eventually forget about them completely. If you really think about it, you will realize that as soon as our enthusiasm diminishes, so does your new habit. Let's face it, most of us aren't enthusiastic about waking up early to go to the gym. I know I certainly wasn't when I first started doing this.

Most of us when we are trying to add a new habit, tend to use the momentum of our excitement to get us started. You may have read a good book that inspired you to run a mile every day, saw an encouraging video online, or saw someone who is in phenomenal shape and you decided to start a new workout plan. Whatever the case may be, most people get extrinsically motivated and rely solely on their enthusiasm to help them develop this new habit. And it works…but he benefits are short lived.

But why is this method only effective in the beginning? You see, our brain likes routines, it likes patterns and habits, because quite frankly they are familiar, they are safe, and they require very little mental energy comparted to trying something new. Even though our brain love routines, they also crave novelty, in other words, our brain likes new things, it loves to learn. I know this sounds like a paradox, but it will make more sense in a little bit. But instead of a paradox, see it as a balance. If our brains are too fixated on routines and patterns, this could be actually become pathological, such as seen in obsessive compulsive disorders (OCD). However, if our brains neglects routines and habits and desires only new stimuli, then that too can be pathological, as in the cases of mania.

Neurologically speaking, our brains are the happiest when we can do both. And this is where we get to the core of my technique on how to develop a new habit. So how do we satisfy both of these seemingly "conflicting" needs?

It is very simple actually, most people are surprised to discover how simple yet effective this technique is. But they almost always become believers once they try it and realize that their success rate for developing a new habit has increases tremendously.

This technique has two parts:

One: add a very small, almost minute, positive habit.

Two: slowly progress in the development of this habit.

This will make a lot more sense with a specific example. So let's say that you have decided that you will run a mile every morning. This is the new habit that you would like to develop. What most people will do is that they will set their alarm early, wake up go for a run, get extremely exhausted and sore, feel miserable and tired and they probably won't run again for another six months. But you are different, because now you know something that they don't. By using this technique, what you will do is set the alarm for waking up a half an hour earlier, and that is it! That is it for the first week! All you are doing is creating new neurological pathways to train your brain to feel comfort in the new "routine" of waking up a half an hour earlier. The beauty of this is that your brain sees this as the perfect balance between "routine" and a "new stimuli". With that extra half an hour, you can do whatever you would like to do, as long as it is not running. I know this sounds complete counter intuitive but trust me, not only have I used this technique with my patients, but I have used it on myself. I used this to wake up at 5:00 am every morning (even on my days off), run a mile, pray, meditate, take a cold shower, and write this book, all before my clinic even opens. This is not to showoff, but rather to act as a testament to how powerful this technique can be if implemented correctly.

Those who have known me for some time, know that I have always been a night owl, even when I was an infant. Yet, I have always longed to be a morning person but I just couldn't do it. Every time I would try, I would fail within three to four days. It wasn't until I realized that I was relying on my just enthusiasm and will power. I wasn't taking advantage of my understanding of my brain's neurological mechanisms, I wasn't putting it to good use. Simply by utilizing this technique, I have been able to develop this healthy habit in less than a month, and I have done it now for quite some time.

Okay, getting back to our example of developing the

habit of running a mile every morning. After about a week or so you will begin to adapt to waking up early, your brain is perfectly comfortable with this new routine. You don't feel any resistance with your new wake up time. At this stage you will continue to wake up a half an hour earlier, like you have been doing but will now introduce a new stimuli; like going outside to walk. Once again, please refrain for going on that mile run at this stage, rather enjoy a nice leisurely walk around your neighborhood. Do this for another week or so, once again, your brain will adapt to this new routine and you will find that if you woke up late and didn't go outside, you will feel like you are missing something. This is a very good sign! At this point this is where you can introduce running into the equation. Again, use the same gradual technique in your running so that you don't overwhelm your brain's habit formation system. Take it easy, have fun, and don't push yourself more than you need to. As one of my mentors, Dr. Mueller, often tells me:

"If you get just 1% better every day, imagine how much better you will be by the end of the year?"

- Dr. Jon Mueller

These gradual yet consistent lifestyle modifications may seem so small that it can be easy to think that they have no benefit what-so-ever. But as you can see, this is actually how our brains are wired to adapt to forming and maintaining new habits. By using this technique you are simultaneously satisfying your brain's need for "routine" and "stimuli".

You will no longer be relying on just motivation, willpower, or an emotional high, but rather you will be using your brain's default setting for establishing new habits. Every habit (whether it is positive or negative) that you have developed from childhood up to this point has been through this exact process, so why are we so adamant about doing it any other way? Any other technique will only produce temporary benefits at best and frustration at worst. By identifying the healthy habits you would like to add into your life and approaching them in this gradual yet effective manner, you will have using a very powerful ally.

The reason this technique is so effective is because the hardest part of any positive change is getting it started. So if you can trick your brain into starting a new habit you have actually done the hardest part. Believe it or not the hardest part of running a mile in the morning from a neurological point of view is the waking up early to accommodate for your run. Unfortunately, what most of us tend to do is set overly ambitious goals, use the sheer power of our excitement and the strength of our willpower to get started and lose motivation and return to our old habits none the wiser. Imagine if this was something we learned from a young age. Who knows, we maybe able to flip that statistics of the failure rate of new year's resolutions from 92% to turning that number into the success rate.

A simple and yet effective example I often give to my patients to illustrate the power of this technique, is to get them to drink a cup of water before each meal. Most of us could benefit from drinking more water. And even though this seems like a very simple habit, the health benefits from doing this are tremendously profound. Not only are they going to be much more hydrated, but the added water primes the digestive tract, preparing it for the consumption of food, thus aiding in digestion.

Another added bonus is that because you have filled your stomach with some water before your meal, you may notice that you eat less food. This is because the added water gives your stomach the sensation of feeling full, faster, which results in more satisfied with eating less food. Over time this little new habit can help you lose extra body fat virtually effortlessly.

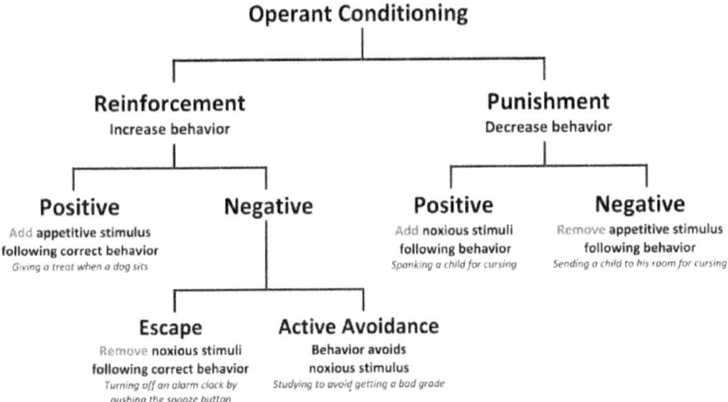

The diagram above is one of the foundational pillars in the field of psychology on behavior modification through reward and punishment. It is still taught and used in many psychology clinics and universities. However, in my humble opinion, I think it still relies too heavily on the use of willpower, and thus the results tend to be temporary except, of course, in extreme cases. If you look at the examples mentioned in the smaller font on the diagram, you can see that for nearly every situation, it is a temporary behavior modification. Take for instance the "turning off the alarm clock by pushing the snooze button" this uses negative reinforcement (the annoying alarm sound) to increase a positive behavior (waking up early). Does this model train us to wake up early on our own, once we have it established? Not likely, as a matter of fact, most people who use an alarm clock to wake up early will rely on it for the rest of their lives. in my opinion that is not an authentic positive change. Sure it is better than nothing, however it lends itself to being more of a crutch than an agent of change.

Or the example of "sending a child to his room for cursing." What that typically does is train the child to not curse in the house/ around the parents, but it doesn't mean that it will permanently eliminate his swearing. If this model was truly effective then behavior modification should be a breeze, yet it is not.

Disclaimer: This is just my humble opinion. I am not a practicing psychologist and thus am not qualified to speak on this topic. The principles mentioned about go against traditional psychological understanding of changing a behavior, so take it with a grain of salt). It is my opinion that our current understanding of adding positive habits and eliminating negative ones is very dated and at best an over simplistic explanation. It fails to address the complexity of the neurological processes and mechanisms in the brain. I believe that this is a very good model for training a pet, but it simply does not deliver lasting results in humans. Before making any lifestyle changes, please talk to your healthcare provider and get their approval first.

The reason I am stating all of this is to let you know that every time you have tried a new diet, a new workout, a new habit, or tried to cut a bad habit and failed. It wasn't due to you being a failure, or weak, or unintelligent. It was rather due to a very dated psychological model that was discovered on animal behavior and then applied to human behavior. And this is very important because if you want to make lasting and effective change, you need to be aware of that. You can't see yourself as a failure, you can't give up hope on yourself, because it wasn't you that was broken, but rather it is the model that we use to change our habits that is broken.

That is why I have worked vigorously to discover and present to you my two principles for changing your behavior. **Principle 1** uses your brain's neurological reward system to eliminate a negative habit while **Principle 2** uses your brain's regulatory and adaptive mechanism to add a positive habit into your life.

What I have found is that most people tend to get much better and longer lasting results when they implement principle 1 and principle 2. Simply by using these two principles, you give yourself the best opportunity to make real, lasting changes in your life.

THE SOLUTION

HOW TO JUMPSTART YOUR BODY'S HEALING

OMEGA-3 FATTY ACIDS

Most of us have heard from one source or another that fish oils are heart healthy, but what we may not have been told is that the health benefits of fish oils far exceed beyond just the heart. It's not really fish oils that are so healthy but the active fatty component in the fish's oil called omega-3, those omega-3s are so incredibly healthy for our bodies. There are a few fundamental aspects of omega-3 that we need to understand before diving into the plethora of their health benefits. That way we can take advantage of their maximum benefits.

For starters, omega-3s are not just found in fish oils, as a matter of fact they can be found in some seeds and nuts too, such as walnuts, chia seeds, and flax seeds. When you break down omega-3s into their molecular form, you will see that there are three types:

- **EPA (eicosapentaenoic acid)**

- **DHA (docosahexaenoic acid)**

- **ALA (alpha-linoleic acid)**

EPA and **DHA** are of marine animal origin. **ALA,** on the other hand, are derived from plants. Marine sources of Omega-3 are much more powerful and effective than plant sources. The reason being is that ALA does have to go through extra conversions in the body before the body can turn it into EPA, which is its more usable form in the body. ALA also requires more enzymes to break it down into its usable form. When you consume your omega-3s from marine origins, your body doesn't have to go through that rigorous conversion process and so it can use the EPA and DHA right away. Thus it is widely accepted and documented that if you can consume omega-3 from marine origins, you will be able to get far greater health benefits than consuming them from plants. This is clearly demonstrated in the flow chart below.

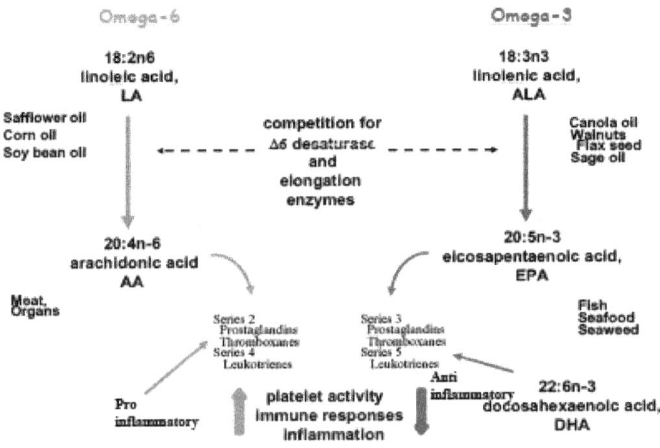

As you may have noticed from the flow chart above, there are two Omegas fatty acids that are essential for the proper functioning of our body, provided that they are consumed in their proper rations. Omega-6 however, plays a different role in the body, while omega-3s are anti-inflammatory, omega-6 are proinflammatory. Upon first learning this, you might think that omega-6s are bad, however, remember inflammation is not a bad thing, it is essential for the body to heal properly. We do need omega-6s in our diet so our bodies can produce the proper immune and inflammatory markers needed to fight pathogens, remove irritants, and rejuvenate damaged cells. Contrary to that, omega-3s are essential for the production of anti-inflammatory markers and hormones that allow the body to turn down that inflammatory process when it is no longer needed, ensuring that we do not enter into a long term state of inflammation (chronic inflammation). You can think of omega-6s and omega-3s as the **"on"** and **"off"** button for inflammation in the body. The key here is to make sure that we consume both in the proper ratio that is optimal for our body's healing processes. Interestingly, these two omega's need the same enzymes to be transformed, absorbed, and used in the body. So if we consume too much omega-6s in our diet, it monopolizes the enzymes that would otherwise be needed to absorb and use omega-3 fatty acids. This can cause our bodies to struggles to observe the little omega-3 that you maybe consuming in your diet already. This opens up a whole world of troubles as far as your health goes.

There are four types of omega-6s, three of which we can naturally produce in our body. However, that leaves one form of omega-6, known as **linoleic acid** which we need to consume since our body cannot create it. Most of us don't have to worry about that since, it is found in abundance in our standard American diet. Contrarily, omega-3s cannot be created in the body, so we need to consume them in our diet. Most of us in the United States are severely deficient in omega-3s. Thus Linoleic acid and Omega-3s are known as **"essential"** fatty acids; because it is essential for us to consume them in our diets.

One of the main contributors for chronic inflammation and all the diseases associated with it is due to the over consumption of omega-6s and the under consumption of omega-3s. Historically our diet has changed a lot in the last 100 years. In the past, the meat that we used to hunt or raise, grazed on grass and seeds. They were able to eat the foods that they were designed to eat and in return that meat was rich in the healthy fats. But now we have industrialized the meat industry so cattle and livestock are raised eating foods that they would never typically eat in nature, such as soy, corn meal, grains and other cheap filler foods. Those foods happened to also be very high in omega-6s, because ironically enough that allows the cattle go get fatter and thus produce more delicious fatty cuts of meat. Consequently, the meat we consume now has a far greater amount of omega-6 than it ever did in the past.

Throughout human history, we had to work hard to hunt or raise livestock. The animals ate what they intuitively wanted to eat, such as grass and hay, allowing their meat to have far less omega-6. Back then meat consumption was typically saved for rare and special occasions. So when people did eat meat, they did so in moderation. This too contributed to far less omega-6 consumption in their diets. But due to the convenience of grocery stores and fast food restaurants, not only are we consuming more meat than ever before, we are eating meats that are very high in omega-6s. Thus we are consuming a far greater amount of omega-6 than our body actually needs which throughs us off the omega-3 to omega-6 ratio, prompting our bodies to be in a state of chronic pro-inflammation.

Additionally, due the industrialization and the intensive breeding, and the easy accessibility to a wide range of foods, it is easier than ever to over eat plants rich in omega-6 **(palm, sunflower, peanut oil, etc.)** Most people in the United States can greatly improve their health if they simply cut down the high omega-6 containing plants, oils, and meats from their diets.

A 100 years ago, our omega-3 to omega-6 ration consumption was **1:3**. Meaning that for every gram of omega-3 we consumed, we would consume 3 grams of omega-6. That is actually very close to the ideal ratio of omega-3 to omega-6 needed to maintain a healthy inflammatory response. That also happens to be the very close to the ratio that humans have had throughout most of our history here on earth. However, currently in the United States, that ratio has become as high as **1:40**. It is no wonder why we are plagued with the diseases caused by chronic inflammation. Our bodies literally can't even produce the required anti-inflammatory hormones with such high levels of omega-6s and low levels of omega-3s. We have turned "on" the inflammatory process and our body does not have the building blocks and necessary nutrients to turn it "off" when it needs to.

Most of us in North American have to make a conscious effort to consume the proper amount of omega-3s. However, that is not the case in other places around the world such as the "Mediterranean" region and the "blue-zones". These areas have the greatest concentration of **centennials** (people who live longer than a 100 years) in the world. The blue-zones are made up of random regions in South America, Greece, japan, and Italy. At first glance, it may seem like these regions have no relationship with each other what-so-ever. Scientists and researchers however, have always been fascinated with those who live there because when they study the locals of those regions, they found that not only do the locals have the highest concentration of centennials but those centennials are active, mentally sharp, and overall very healthy. They have a high quality of life, most of them aren't bed ridden, or on life support, or bound to a wheel chair. This absolutely baffled researchers and they began funding large amounts of research to see what those regions all have in common. One of the common threads between all of them was that they consume a far greater number of omega-3s than we do. And that their overall omega-3 to omega-6 ratios are a lot closer to what our bodies need to have a healthy inflammatory process.

Scientific evidence has consistently shown that deficiency in omega-3 can lead to cardiovascular disease and a host of brain diseases ranging from depression, attention deficit, Alzheimer's disease, stroke, and even Parkinson's. Even though there isn't enough research to show what the exact doses of omega-3s are necessary to actually **"prevent"** a disease, one thing is certain, there are numerous studies that show that marine based omega-3s of the EPA and DHA have significant benefits for virtually every system in our body. Their properties gives them a wide range of protective and curative effects on many diseases and ailments. Let's dive into how your body uses omega-3's to produce such profound anti-inflammatory health benefits.

OMEGA-3S AND INFLAMMATION

Recently, the anti-inflammatory effects of omega-3 fatty acids have attracted a lot of attention in the scientific community. They found that all our cell contain significant amounts of fatty acids. The fatty acids are actually essential for the cell to have proper integrity and cellular communication with the other cells in the body. Healthy fats such as omega-3s allow the cells membrane (the border of each cell) to be healthy and flexible allowing proper nutrients to enter into the cell. They do this by reducing a very powerful inflammatory marker called **arachidonic acid (AA)** which hardens and damages the cell border. Since high omega-6 consumption increases arachidonic acid (AA), this leads the cell border to harden and become ridged, which restricts the cell's ability to absorb nutrients. A cell that is unable to absorb the essential nutrients it needs to function, becomes dysfunctional and typically has a shorter life span. Of course this automatically leads to the cell triggering an inflammatory response, in hopes that the inflammation will rejuvenate and heal the cell border. If this were to happen in the cells of your heart, over a long period of time, you would have unhealthy heart cells, which eventually will lead to those cells dying pre-maturely and the remaining heart cells not functioning properly. I think we both know what that could lead to if not properly addressed. So this is an important thing to remember as you go through your health journey.

Just as I have mentioned in the earlier chapter of **"The Healing Ratio"**, to maximize the health benefits of omega-3, we first have to reduce the amount of omega-6 foods that we are eating and then add the high omega-3 foods into our diet. Even if we were to increase our omega-3 consumption, most of the enzymes that we need to absorb and use those omega-3s will be used by the omega-6s that you are consuming. By reducing the omega-6s that you are consuming in your diet, you free up some of these essential enzymes so that they can work with the omega-3s and promote the anti-inflammatory benefits that you are looking for.

Interestingly the EPA and DHA that make up the omega-3 fatty acids have different effects on different body parts. DHA provides powerful brain health benefits, while the EPA reduces chronic inflammation (the source of almost all age-related diseases in the United States).

Amazingly, omega-3s have been shown to activate the transcription of certain genes that improve inflammation, meaning that regular omega-3 consumption can quite literally change your genetic coding for how your body responds to inflammation. Thus making your body's ability to fight pathogens, remove irritants, and rejuvenate damaged cells more effective and better at being able to regulate itself to the healthy range, making it far less likely for you to be in a chronically inflammated state.

OMEGA-3S AND THE CARDIOVASCULAR SYSTEM

The cardio-protective effects of omega-3 fatty acids still continue to impresses researchers and doctors to this very day. Sadly, the majority of us in the United States are at risk of having a high level of harmful blood lipids. The proportion of good and bad cholesterol is a very powerful predictor as to whether one is more likely to have cardiovascular disease or not. We have commonly been told that cholesterol is the chief lipid that is absolutely to be avoided if we want to avoid vascular diseases such heart disease and stroke.

Ironically enough, cholesterol is something that your body can naturally produce, and it usually does so to reduce inflammation, regulate proper hormone production, promote neuronal growth, and it's even essential for our body's ability to produce and absorb vitamin D. Often times, having high cholesterol is a sign that your body is trying to reduce inflammation. Initially doctors thought that having elevated cholesterol is what causes heart disease, however, the more accurate way of looking at this is that having high cholesterol is your body's way of trying to reduce chronic inflammation. The longer your cholesterol levels are elevated the more chronic your inflammation is, and thus are more likely to suffer from heart disease. Simply trying to reduce our cholesterol is not enough to reducing our risk of heart disease, because doing so is not getting to the root of the matter. It is much more advisable to see why our body is producing such high levels of cholesterol and treat that, instead of just trying to lower your cholesterol levels.

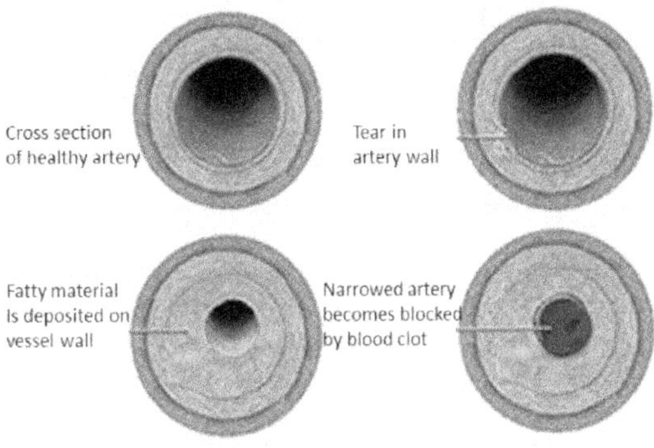

It is important to note that there is good cholesterol HDL (which actually protects against heart disease) and bad cholesterol (called LDL). What Omega-3s do really well is that they help stabilize the relationship between good and bad cholesterol by lowering the ratio of bad cholesterol. Omega-3 fatty acids decrease the assembly and secretion of this very bad cholesterol and they help our cells use fat for cellular energy thus resulting in lower blood triglyceride levels. Lower blood triglycerides, therefore means that there is a lower development of plaque buildup on the artery (atherosclerosis) and thus prevent the formation of clots in the blood that can block blood vessels in the heart, brain, or lungs; they therefore have been shown to directly reduce the risk of strokes, heart attacks, and even pulmonary embolisms.

As demonstrated in the image in the above, having

cholesterol and fats circulating in our blood for many years can eventually lead to plaque buildup, reducing the amount of blood that can travel to that region. If it is sever enough the whole blood vessel can be blocked. This is something we want to avoid at all costs.

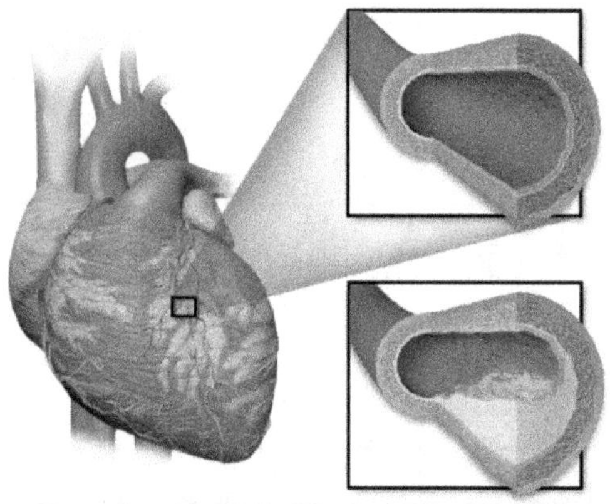

Normal and Partially Blocked Blood Vessels

Omega-3s also protect the lining of arteries, allowing them to be strong and flexible so that the heart doesn't have to work as hard to pump blood to the rest of your body. This is also the mechanism by which they can lower blood pressure. By allowing the blood vessels to relax, the pressure of the blood vessels decrease, thus lowering the risk of high blood pressure and dangerous risks of bursting an artery.

A nice little side bonus of omega-3s is that they are

well-known to reverse the effects on **insulin resistance**. Remember all the negative signs and symptoms that can manifest from insulin resistance in the body? Of courses we can't just rely on omega-3 to help us with insulin resistance; it is important to make a conscious effort to lower processed carbohydrates and sugar consumption, but omega-3s can totally complement that lifestyle change too. In 2014, a natural molecule derived from omega-3 was discovered by researchers from Quebec Faculty of Medicine of Laval University. This molecule was shown to have beneficial effects on insulin resistance and treatment of type 2 diabetes and its effects were even comparable to those of some pharmaceutical drugs. That's pretty remarkable, when you consider how easy it is to consume more omega-3s in your diet.

OMEGA-3S AND PSYCHOLOGICAL DISORDERS

Healthy fats are essential to the normal functioning of the brain and the nervous system. This makes a lot more sense when you consider the fact that more than 60% of our brain is fat; more specifically it is mostly composed of DHA(docosahexaenoic acid) omega-3 fat.

For this and many other reasons omega-3 fatty

acids work as allies to the brain. They help fight depression, memory problems, Alzheimer's disease and Attention Deficit / Hyperactivity Disorder (ADHD). Many reports clearly show the benefits of omega-3s on the nervous system, by increasing the number of neurotransmitters while ensuring proper function of the neurons that are already there. That is what I call a "win-win situation".

Sadly most of us at one point or another have experienced or will experience depression and/or anxiety. Both of these are complex mood disorders that can have many different triggers. But scientists are now referring to depression and anxiety as "inflammation of the Brain". Interestingly, more and more studies have linked mood disorders not just the inflammation in the brain but also to Omega-3 deficiencies. We now know that the combination of chronic inflammation and the imbalance of omega-3 consumption play a very direct role with these and many other mood disorders.

Omega-3s help fight against anxiety, stress and depression through many different mechanisms. Omega-3s EPA and DHA, once transformed in the body, can increase prostaglandin derivatives. These have anti-inflammatory properties throughout the whole body, not just the brain and nervous system. They accelerate the transmission of nerve impulses, and improve the growth and plasticity of nerve cells. This is very important, because if the neurons in the brain are having a hard time communicating with each other, it is going to be hard for the brain to be excited and stimulated. That is one of the hallmarks we see with depression, they lose their ability to enjoy the activities they once loved, and their overall enthusiasm for life. We want the neurons to be able to communicate with each other smoothly. Additionally, we want them to be able grow and be able to adapt to life's various stimuli and situations. When our neurons aren't allowed to grow and adapt, we see that it can cause that "stuck" feeling. This is very common with people who suffer from depression, they know what they must do, but they can't because they feel stuck. Very simply, from a neurological point of view, omega-3s can potentially help with becoming unstuck.

It is pretty widely accepted that omega-3s may be a good addition to people who respond poorly to antidepressant drugs. Of course it is vital that you speak to your healthcare provider before adding or subtracting anything to your current medications.

Thankfully the benefits of omega-3s don't stop

there, since there is more and more evidence suggesting that they can help protect the brain against dementia, memory loss, and impaired cognitive abilities. These positive effects are noticed in people with progressive memory loss associated with aging; and to potentially slow down the progression of Alzheimer's disease. Interestingly the same mechanism that omega-3 can help with potentially treating depression and anxiety are the same ways they can help slow down the progression of Alzheimer's disease and age related memory loss. When it comes to brain health, good transmission of nerve impulses and neurons and neuron plasticity and growth are the name of the game!

SOURCES OF OMEGA-3

If there is no history of heart failure and you have been cleared with your primary healthcare physician, the recommendations are to consume fatty fish at least twice a week in addition to consuming plant foods rich in ALA such as walnuts, chia seeds, flax seeds, etc.

If, for one reason or another, you cannot consume these foods or consume enough of them, it is possible to take fatty acid supplements in the form of capsules or oil. Of course deriving it from whole foods is the best option, but I understand not everyone loves seafood, or has access to high quality fish. **Unfortunately, here in the United States, it can be quite difficult to consume enough omega-3 through our modern diet alone**. In this case, supplementing with omega-3s are the second best option. If you are going to be supplementing with omega-3s you should be aware that not all fish oils supplements are created equal. There is a lot of irregularity in the manufacturing, testing, sourcing, and packaging of fish oils.

When looking at an omega-3 supplement, pay close attention to the dosage of EPA and DHA, as each one has it own set of health properties. Depending on your needs you can find a supplement with higher DHA dosage or EPA. Most Omega-3 capsules contain fish oils derived from sardine, mackerel and/or anchovy oils, but even that can vary widely from manufacturer to manufacturer.

Generally speaking, it is recommended to start the dosing with omega-3 supplements at 1000 mg per day or 1 gram. That is a great dose to build a powerful anti-inflammatory foundation. If you are advised to increase your dose, then gradually increase it another 1000 mg per day, however do not exceed 4000 mg per day. It is a good idea to start off with the 1000 mg dose and then after a month or two, you can increase it by another 1000 mg. omega-3s have a natural blood thinning effect in the body, which also attributes to its positive cardiovascular effects. But for that reason, it is important to note that if you are already taking anything that has blood thinning properties such aspirin or blood thinning medication, to get the approval from your health care provider.

The general recommended dosage can change depending on the state of your health and how much omega-3s you are consuming from your diet. Consult your doctor, who can guide you in the ideal dosage according to your health status and needs.

I've had many people voice their concern about the fish oil turning rancid. That is a very good thing to be aware of and usually applies to omega-3s that are not thoroughly extracted or are potentially contaminated. Oil and fats in general have a very long shelf life, and if you get a omega-3 fish oil supplement that is high quality and tested during the extraction and packaging process, then chances are you don't have to worry about that. That is why a quality supplement is very important. To illustrate how important a quality supplement is, I would personally rather have you not taking a fish oil product than taking a low-grade supplement. But with that being said, taking a high quality product can make all the difference in our health. So how can we find a high quality omega-3 supplement?

When it comes to quality, there are a few things to keep in mind to ensure that you are getting the best product on the market. One of the most important characteristic of a high quality omega-3 product is the source of fish in which they extract the omega-3 fatty acids. Of course we want healthy, fatty, wild fish that is either from the ocean or the sea. Consuming fish oil from farm raised fish is a big no-no. Farm raised fish are essentially fish that are raised in large pool, they manually fed by their farmers and generally don't have enough space to swim around freely. The problem here is that these fish excrete their waste in this pool and some of them die in this pool and it is very easy for disease and bacteria to contaminate the fish. This is not where we want our omega-3s to be extracted from. What we want are fish that swim freely in clean ocean/sea waters, that eat the foods that they instinctually eat to ensure that they have the highest quality of omega-3 fatty acids.

Another concern is the contamination of heavy metals such as mercury in the fish oils. There are two things to be aware of to ensure that you are consuming omega-3 with minimal risk of mercury exposure. The first thing is see if the supplement comes from "pelagic fish". This is a very important characteristic of a high quality fish oil, that sadly not too many people are aware off. Imagine the sea is separated into three layers; the top one third layer on the surface of the water, the middle layer, and then the lower one third layer which is on the sea floor. Ideally we want fish that lives in the middle layer of the sea/ocean, those are the fish that are classified as the "pelagic fish".

The reason this is essential is because, there are a lot of human waste and contamination such as oils, chemicals, and plastics that naturally raise to the top layer of the sea/ocean waters. Likewise, there is a lot of heavy metals, rust, and human waste products that sink to the bottom of the sea/ocean. Fish that primarily live in the top layer or the bottom layer of the sea are not usually the highest quality because they spend all their lives in potentially unclean waters and could be exposed to things that pelagic fish typically would not be exposed to.

Of course, the other factor that is vital to ensuring a pure omega-3 supplement is that fish oil is filtered and is third-party tested for impurities, contaminants, heavy metals, bacteria, etc. A company that is willing to spend the extra money to have an independent third party company test and check their fish oil products for impurities, is a company that really cares about their customers' health.

Characteristics of a high quality fish oil supplement

-Harvested from the ocean/sea

-Extracted from pelagic fish to minimize environmental contaminations

-Avoid fish oil from farm raised fish

-3rd party tested for contamination, heavy metals, bacteria, fungi, impurities, etc.

-At least 500mg of actual omega-3 per serving

Dosage for Omega-3

Cardiovascular Benefits:

- Preventative dosage: 1000 mg total of EPA and DHA per day.

- Intervention (if you are already at risk of a cardiovascular condition): Up to 2000 mg total of EPA and DHA per day.

- Decrease inflammation: Between 2400 mg to 4000 mg total of EPA and DHA per day.

Nervous System/Psychological Benefits:

- Adolescent with ADHD (Attention Deficit Disorder with Hyperactivity): 2000 mg total of EPA and DHA with a minimum of 400 mg DHA per day.

- Depression: 4000 mg to 9000 mg total of EPA and DHA per day.

- Memory and cognitive decline: 3000 mg total of EPA and DHA, with a minimum of 1000 mg DHA per day.

***Disclaimer:** Again, please check with your health care provider before taking any supplements and/or changing your diet. The dosage mentioned in this book are general guidelines and are considered high dosages. Omega-3 fatty acids naturally have a blood thinning effect. This actually attributes to some of its cardiovascular benefits, but can cause side-effects for certain people. If you are on blood thinners, aspirin, and/or certain medications and supplements, please talk to your doctor before increasing omega-3/seafood consumption. Likewise, if you have a blood disorder, please let your primary doctor know before taking omega-3 fatty acids or increasing seafood consumption.

TURMERIC

This special root originally from India, has been used for its health benefits for well over a millennia. Even the ancient writings of explorer Marco Polo mention this golden yellow spice dating as far back as 1290 AD. Its description and health benefits have been documented in various writings dating back to even further than that. It has been very popular in the east and it continues to gain popularity due to its versatile use. The people of India and various parts of Asia have been using it not only as a spice but as medicine for its ability to both prevent diseases and cure them. Even though its health benefits have been recognized for centuries, it is only recently that we started researching and using it here in the United States.

Through the centuries, there have been many health benefits attributed to this golden root, much of which make it seem too good to be true. Claims such as:

- Curing/preventing certain cancers
- Removing toxins from the blood

- Relieving depression

- Slowing down the progression of Alzheimer's

- Aids with digestion

- Easing arthritis pain and discomfort

- Improves joint mobility and flexibility

- Reduces inflammation

But what are the true benefits of this oriental root whose mysteries are only recently being discovered by science? Which of these claims are actually true, and which are purely an exaggeration? During the time of writing this book, there have been over 6,000 studies done on turmeric and its main active molecule known as curcumin. And just to diffuse the suspense; yes, all the health benefits mentioned above are born of evidence.

Many people may have heard the words Curcumin and turmeric used interchangeably, however there is a big difference. Curcumin is the active compound in turmeric root. Curcumin makes up anywhere between 5% to 9% of the turmeric root, it is universally accepted that curcumin is the most powerful component of turmeric. However, from my clinical experience, I have found that there are many other compounds that are naturally found in turmeric that work synergistically together to provide you with the optimal health benefits. Compounds such as essential oils, omega-3 fatty acids, phytonutrients, antioxidants, etc.

With such a large number of emerging studies in the last decade, even the FDA is beginning to recognize that the active compound curcumin has positive digestive properties such as allowing the food to go through the digestive track more effectively, thus allowing you to be able to absorb more nutrients from the food that you do eat. Turmeric's ability to help in nearly every aspect of the digestive system is another reason why I recommend it for those who have leaky gut syndrome.

HOW CURCUMIN REDUCES INFLAMMATION

So what is the big deal with turmeric and how does it work to reduce chronic inflammation? Based on what the research has shown us, it appears that curcumin has a very unique property on the body. When consumed, curcumin actually binds with different parts of our DNA that are in charge of cellular replication and repair. Thus turning on various gene signals for modulating growth factors. So what does this mean in English? It means that curcumin can actually speed up your body's natural healing factors. Additionally, it can improve your body's ability to make new, healthy, functional cells.

Not only is this absolutely remarkable, but the best part is that is not the only mechanism of healing that it has. Curcumin also modifies certain parts of our immune system known as cytokines, which are directly in charge of the inflammatory response in the body. What this does is it helps our body return to a healthy, normal inflammatory response and can actually prevent the development of diseases associated with prolonged (chronic) inflammation.

As demonstrated in the image on the below, when your body produces too much cytokines, your inflammatory response increases. The curcumin molecule directly gets involved in that pathway and reduces inflammation.

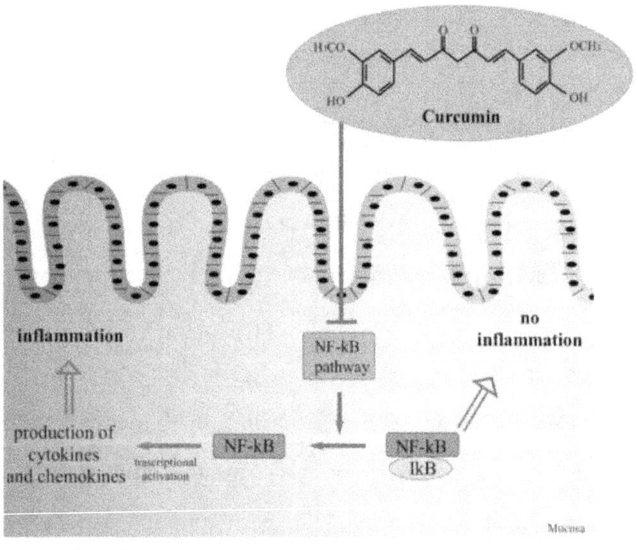

It is then no surprise that curcumin has natural anti-inflammatory properties comparable to non-steroidal anti-inflammatory drugs (NSAIDs). As a matter of fact, some studies have shown curcumin to be more powerful than the commonly taken ibuprofen! And The best part is that the way curcumin works in the body to reduce inflammation is so natural that it does not come with the potential side-effects that other anti-inflammatory drugs and over-the-counters have.

I know many of my patients think that taking over the counter anti-inflammatory medications such as Advil® and Motrin® (and other NSAIDs) are completely safe. I know many people who carry NSAIDs in their purse, store them in their car, have them in a drawer at work, or right next to them in bed for daily use.

This may come as a surprise, but consider this, the FDA has estimated that there are at least 16,000 deaths per year in the United States directly caused by using NSAIDs, and a whopping 100,000 people sent to the emergency room due to NSAID related health complications. Prolonged use of NSAIDs can tax the kidneys and liver, cause internal bleeding, ulcers, and many other health issues. Just because it is something that you can buy without a prescription, doesn't necessarily mean that it won't come with negative side-effects.

I don't want to alarm you or make you shy away from ever taking these products. As it is important to note that most of these statistics apply to people who are using NSAIDs on a regular bases. And guess why they are using these anti-inflammatory drugs for long periods of time? Because they have chronic inflammation.

Interestingly, for all of you who have a scientific background. Curcumin reduces the three primary inflammatory markers in the body. It reduces the enzyme Cyclooxygenase II, which is an enzyme responsible for inflammation and pain. It reduces the LOX-2 enzyme which is another pro-inflammatory enzyme. And of course, as mentioned earlier, curcumin modulates the cytokine pathway which is the immune systems response to inflammation, making sure that our inflammatory response doesn't go haywire or go on for longer than it needs to.

Curcumin does something that is also very vital for reducing chronic inflammation. Remember in the chapter, where I discussed the negative effects of free radicals, which damage our healthy cells, and makes them much more susceptible to disease, dysfunction, and early cellular death? This, in return, promotes chronic inflammation even further. The damage done by those free radicals is known as oxidative damage. Thus we need anti-oxidants to protect the cells from this oxidative stress and the damage done from free radicals. That is why you may have heard so much about the benefits of anti-oxidants when it comes to preventative health.

Many of the active compounds found in turmeric, including curcumin, have powerful antioxidant properties. The main mechanism by which the compounds found in turmeric protect the body from oxidative damage is by boosting glutathione, which is our body's main protector against free radicals. Glutathione then scavenges for those free radicals in the body and eliminates them, thus they don't even have a chance to cause oxidative stress to our cells. This is one of the ways in which the body protects itself by preventing damage from happening in the first place. Turmeric also strengthens the outer barriers of our cells thus making them more resilient against the damage done by free radicals.

CLINICAL BENEFITS OF TURMERIC

Thankfully the benefits of turmeric don't top there; due to its versatile anti-inflammatory, anti-oxidant, and rejuvenative properties, turmeric can positively affect virtually every system in the body. It has been proven to protect the body from very diverse diseases, below are some of the most common ones.

ARTHRITIS

One of the most common reasons people use turmeric is for its ability to reduce inflammation in the joints. In a randomized study of a group of patients with rheumatoid arthritis, some people received either curcumin or a NSAID known as phenylbutazone for a period of 2 weeks. At the end of those two weeks, the study found that those who received curcumin showed **the same amount of symptom improvement** as the anti-inflammatory group, but with less side effects! There was a significant reduction of symptoms such as morning joint stiffness, decreased joint swelling, and a reduction in pain.

This is just one of many human studies that validate turmeric's benefits on reducing joint inflammation and the symptoms associated with it. Those are people who could have potentially been taking NSAIDs for the rest of their lives, just to try to get relief from their joint pain and stiffness.

SKIN IRRITATION

Because the compounds found in turmeric are anti-inflammatory and have an anti-irritating effect, historically and even to this day, people have placed turmeric root on cuts, wounds, rashes, and even acne to sooth and disinfect the area.

In one recent study done on patients with psoriasis lesions, a group of 10 people with psoriasis were asked to rub turmeric ointment on the affected area. Five out of the ten of these individuals saw 90% reduction of skin lesions between 2 to 6 weeks, and 5 others had seen their lesions regress from 50% to 85% after 8 weeks. It is also an excellent way to purify the scalp and rid of problems such as dandruff, itching and eczema.

It is proven that curcumin can also slow hair loss as it helps to activate blood circulation to the scalp and increase that growth factor we had talked about earlier. One of the benefits of the increased growth factor is that it plays a positive role reducing the death of hair follicles, thus reducing hair loss.

DIGESTIVE DISEASE

Turmeric has traditionally been used to relieve a wide

range of digestive disorders, such as nausea, heaviness, indigestion, leaky gut syndrome, stomach pain, and bloating. Many people even use it after eating too much, as it is excellent at healing and soothing the digestive tract. The way turmeric is able to help in such a wide range of digestive ailments is due to the fact that it helps your body release the appropriate amount of stomach acid and bile. These are two secretion that your body releases when you eat a meal. They are essential for your ability to break down the food that you ate into small enough pieces so that your body can use it for energy. Of course producing too much or too little stomach acid and bile can be problematic.

The consumption of turmeric has shown in studies to do something very amazing. For those who produce too much stomach acids, it helps them produce less; while for those who produce too little stomach acids, it helps them produce more. It does the same things with bile production, which helps break down the fats that we eat. In other words, it balances out your digestive secretions based on your imbalances. That is quite extraordinary considering that turmeric acts as a customizable healer based on your body's digestive weakness. It helps regulate and bring these digestive secretions back to healthy levels.

It is no surprise that even the World Health

Organization has recognized its ability to aid in treating gastric ulcers, diarrhea, and even help those who produce too much stomach acids and need to take anti-acids.

CANCER

One of the most incredible therapeutic benefits of turmeric is in its anti-carcinogenic effects; primarily because turmeric has both anti-oxidant and anti-inflammatory effects on the body. According to research, this combination leads to a synergistic effect on the prevention and treatment of certain cancers.

I know this may sound frightening, but the reality is that at any given time, a healthy body can technically have cancer cells. The reason, however, we don't all develop cancer is because the body is able to detect these cancerous cells and signals them to be aborted. This facilitated programed cellular death is called apoptosis. Our body is constantly forming new cells and getting rid of dysfunctional, cancerous cells. When someone develops diagnosable cancer, the mechanism of apoptosis (programed cellular death) doesn't work properly. And so the cancer cells grow and grow, till they spread to nearby cells, tissues, then organs.

For example, those with a tongue cancer lesion saw a

10% reduction in the size of this cancerous lesion with the use of a topical turmeric agent.

Curcumin also demonstrates anti-cancer benefits by encouraging the body to recognize and trigger cellular death of cancer cells. This situation has been observed in different types of cancer, including:

- Lung cancer

- Pancreas cancer

- Ovarian cancer

- Colon cancer

Interestingly, those cancers tend to be less common in Asian countries where turmeric is consumed as a regular part of their cuisine. Because of its amazing abilities, it is not surprising that curcumin is being examined as a potential cancer prevention agent. Of course, nothing is a hundred percent guaranteed, but the evidence seems to be quite encouraging.

TURMERIC PRE-CAUTIONS

Thankfully, with all these mentioned health benefits, turmeric is generally recognized as safe ingredient and supplement. However, it does act as a natural blood thinner, so it is not recommended with those with blood disorders, on blood thinning medication, or to take within two weeks of surgery. Please talk with your doctor before adding turmeric or curcumin in your diet or supplementation regimen. Here are some specific situations that require extra attention before using turmeric:

- Do not use a turmeric/curcumin supplement when **pregnant or breast feeding**.
- Those with **gallbladder stones or gallbladder** problems might find that turmeric exacerbates them.
- Those who are on **blood thinners/anticoagulant drugs.**
- Turmeric may slow blood clotting, so those with **bleeding problems and/or an upcoming surgery** should not take it.
- Curcumin might decrease blood sugar in **diabetics**.
- High amounts of turmeric might affect **iron absorption.**
- Too much turmeric consumption might increase the production of stomach acid, which could be problematic for those with **reflux or ulcers.**

In 2001, a study on the safety of turmeric in humans was performed, the results of the study concluded that in general most people can take a dose range from 500 mg to 8000 mg of turmeric root daily for a period of 3 months without any relative toxicity. The dosages of 500 mg to 8,000 mg of turmeric per day may seem high, but keep in mind that this is the actual whole root. It is not the extracted or supplemented dose. Most supplements will have extracted the active ingredient in turmeric, so the dosage is generally much smaller (approximately in the range of 250 mg to 2,000 mg). Ideally, if my patient is cleared to take a turmeric supplement, I recommend that they find one with both the extracted curcumin and with the whole turmeric root in there as well; that way they can get all the extra phytonutrients from the whole turmeric root to help the body absorb and utilize the curcuminoids.

Generally speaking though, if the list above does not apply to you and you have had clearance from your doctor, most of us could reap great benefits by increasing our regular turmeric consumption.

PROBIOTICS

There has been a lot of buzz surrounding probiotics lately, and rightfully so.   Before I get into why these little guys have earned the positive propaganda. I would like to talk about what they are so that we understand the significant role they play in our health and how they can help us in the fight against chronic inflammation.

Probiotics are good bacteria that can be found abundantly in our digestive tract. I know it can be a strange notion to learn that there are good bacteria that reside inside of our body. And it maybe even stranger to learn that **there are more bacteria in our body than actual human cells.** I remember when I first learned that, I was shocked. If that disturbs you, I want you to know that without theses good bacteria, we wouldn't survive for very long.

These little bacteria are essential for our ability to break down food and nutrients so that our body can use them. Not only that, but some of these good bacteria release nutrients that are vital for our bodies to function properly. We have a symbiotic relationship with them, meaning, that they benefit from living inside us and we benefit from them too. It is a win-win situation.

What may come as a surprise to you is that probiotics are not just essential for the breakdown of the foods that we eat, so that our bodies can absorbed the vital nutrients, but that they also help you fight the bad bacteria, such as the ones that cause yeast infections, candida, E. coli, etc. The way that they do it, however, is very different than how our immune system fights these pathogens. The best way to explain it is with the following analogy.

Imagine that you got invited to a house party, as soon as you arrive, you find that the house is packed with people that have completely different interests from you. The music playing in the back ground is rough and unpleasant, the place is a mess, and it is crowded and humid. You are just uncomfortable and miserable. I know this sounds pretty horrible, but bear with me. Chances are you would be so uncomfortable in this environment and the type of crowd there, that you would just leave. That is exactly what happens inside our digestive system, well maybe not exactly, but very closely. By having the right amounts of probiotics in our digestive tract, we don't give a chance for the bad bacteria to over grow, spread and take over. The good bacteria overcrowds them and doesn't allow the bad bacteria to go anywhere they are not supposed to.

Since we have a symbiotic relationship with these good bacteria, the foods that we eat literally feeds the bacteria in our gut. So if we are eating healthy, whole foods we will be feeding and creating an environment for the good gut bacteria to thrive. However, if we eat a lot of sugar, gluten, and processed foods, then we will primarily be feeding the bad bacteria in our gut and thus be creating an environment that's favorable for the growth of the bad bacteria. And guess what, the most recent literature has shown that your cravings can, to a very large degree, be effected by the type of bacteria you primarily have in your digestive tract.

Let me reiterate that, if you are primarily feeding the bad bacteria in your gut with sugars, gluten, and processed foods, you will be creating the optimal environment for them to flourish. That will directly play a role in the amount of nutrients that your body can break down, absorb, and use. The bad bacteria, on the other hand, will interfere with that process, thus leading to deficiencies in essential vitamins, minerals, and nutrients needed by your body to be healthy.

Since your body is incredibly intelligent, it begins to recognize that its nutritional needs are not being met, so to fix that problem, your brain begins to release more of the hunger hormones and neurotransmitters so that you can eat more food, and hopefully have a better chance of consuming the essential vitamins and minerals. If we have a habit of eating junk food then we will continue to do so. Then when we get hungry, we will consume more junk food, which will continue to feed those bad bacteria. This becomes a vicious downward spiral.

It is primarily through this mechanism that we have now understood how your gut bacteria can literally alter your cravings to consume the very thing things they need to survive. Have you ever tried pure green leafy vegetable juice and thought that it tasted like grass and you wondered how people actually enjoy drinking this on a regular basis? And do you know that healthy person who no matter how much delicious, unhealthy food you may offer them, they just seem to not really crave it? People eat according to what their gut bacteria need to flourish. What I often see in my clinic is that a patient will come in mentioning that they have a "sweet tooth", they are always craving sweets; they consume a lot of sugar, soda, candy, cake, deserts, etc. No matter how hard they try, that sugar craving doesn't seem to go away, as a matter of fact, it actually seems to gets stronger and stronger with time. They come to me recognizing that this habit is getting out of hand. All the sugar they are consuming is not only causing the rise and fall of insulin, triggering an inflammatory response throughout the body, but is also creating the perfect environment for the bad bacteria to thrive. Thus they multiply and colonize, and begin to effect the release of certain hormones such as those in charge of cravings and hunger, making you much more likely to continue to feed them.

When we eat the wrong foods for long enough, the bad bacteria end up overcrowding the good bacteria in our gut, and this is where we see a lot of health issues begin to manifest. This cycle goes on and on and on, until you consciously recognize it and decide to break it.

By this point I think you are starting to recognize a pattern here. The good bacteria's in our digestive tract play such an essential part for our body's ability to function, they are essential not just for our survival, but for our thriving. Yet most people don't know just how important it is to take care of this delicate eco system that dwells in our gut. As demonstrated in the image below, the good bacteria (in blue) .

How Probiotics Work

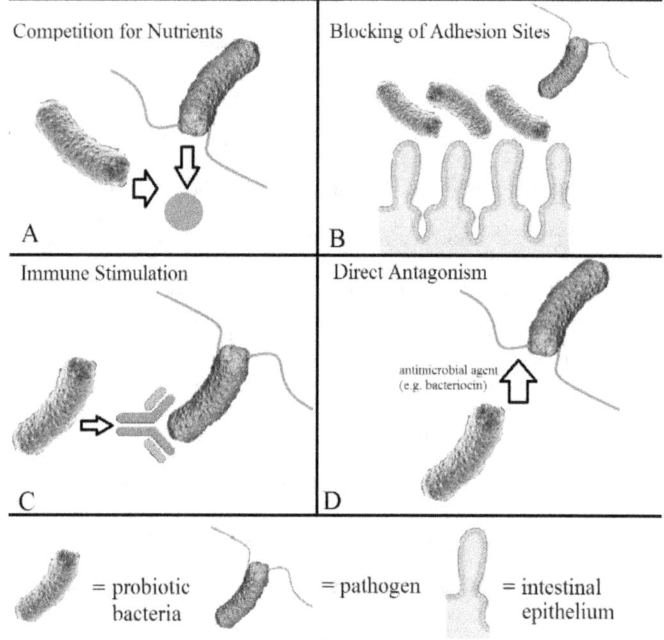

By following all the material in this book, by reducing your sugar, carbohydrate, and gluten consumption, you will be starving the bad bacteria and reducing your chronic inflammation. You will be on the path of healing!

BOOK SUMMERY AND CHEAT SHEET

YOUR QUICK GUIDE TO USING THE MATERIAL IN THIS BOOK

Causes of Chronic Inflammation

- **A Pro-Inflammatory Diet-** Many foods have been called pro-inflammatory. These include especially sugar, unsaturated fats, simple carbohydrates and some oils. A poor omega-3 / omega-6 ratio has also been identified as a factor promoting inflammation

- **Imbalance of Intestinal Flora-** Our intestines are colonized by good bacteria, which help maintain our health. For many reasons (antibiotics, for example), our good bacteria can decrease and leave more room for bad bacteria, which causes several intestinal problems, including permeable walls ("leaky gut") allowing the passage molecules that are harmful to the body. This dysbiosis also favors local inflammation, as in the case in Crohn's disease.

- **Gluten Sensitivity-** Gluten containing foods are most likely to cause food intolerance. When we consume a food that we are intolerant of, the immune system reacts and triggers the inflammatory process considering this food as a foreign body. The same way, toxins that are found in food or the environment, such as pesticides, air pollution, endocrine disruptors, perfumes or food additives, accumulate and stimulate the immune system, which keeps the body reagent permanently.

- **Tobacco / Alcohol / Drugs-** These substances are harmful to health and also promote a chronic inflammatory state.

- **Psychological Stress-** Psychological stress can come in the form of a panic attack and is manifested by a rapid pulse, night sweats and uncontrollable agitation. This is a sign of activity of the hormone called cortisol. Cortisol is (with adrenaline) the hormone responsible for your "fight or protection response". This reaction begins with stimulation of the adrenal glands in response to internal stress. This results in a constriction of the blood vessels, which forces the blood towards the organs in preparation for the stress response. This response becomes a normal state during periods of persistent stress, and chronic inflammation occurs when the immune system and the adrenal glands are over stimulated. This leads to many bad effects on different organs. In the same context, lack of restorative sleep (all phases of which are respected) has been shown to increase cytokine and cortisol levels and maintain chronic pain.

- **Insulin Resistance-** The medical community has also linked insulin and glucose levels to chronic inflammation. For example, obese people who are prone to developing type II diabetes often have problems with chronic inflammation. In the same way, sitting more than eight hours a day increases the chances of developing type II diabetes by 90%. This means that a sedentary lifestyle increases insulin resistance, one of the main factors causing inflammation.

The Effects of Chronic Inflammation:

- **On The Cardiovascular System**- If a high level of bad cholesterol in the blood increases the risk of cardiovascular disease, it does not explain it alone. How is it that half of heart attacks occur in people who have normal or low cholesterol? Although present in small amounts, the cholesterol that adheres to the walls of blood vessels attracts mediators of inflammation. In a person whose inflammation is stimulated excessively, plaques form more easily. Over time, they may create a clot, increasing the chances of heart attack and stroke.

- **Cancerous Cells**- Another discovery of impact, this time for cancerous diseases: the pro-cancerous agents, like the chemicals, the ultraviolet rays or certain infections, would cause cancer by stimulating the inflammatory mechanisms which favor the alterations of the

DNA. For example, some substances released by immune cells during inflammation, such as free radicals, would help them become immortal.

- **Diabetes-** Inflammatory processes would also be directly related to type II diabetes. Currently, it is known that people who have a high degree of inflammation markers (C-reactive protein, interleukin-6) in the blood have an increased risk of developing diabetes. These mediators interfere with the signals of insulin, which gradually prevents cells from absorbing blood sugar. The fat cells would also produce mediators of inflammation, with increased production in case of obesity.

- **Alzheimer Disease-** Stress, especially when it is chronic, has been associated with an increase in inflammatory markers in the blood. It causes a chemical imbalance of the body in addition to promoting the oxidation and the production of free radicals. This mechanism is most often incriminated in the causality of chronic inflammation in the onset of Alzheimer's disease.

- **Depression and Anxiety-** Chronic inflammation of our tissues and organs affects the chemistry of our brain and causes changes in our thoughts, moods and emotions. Let us add that internal inflammation can manifest in many other ways, for example by irritability, or by a sexual dysfunction in men.

Benefits of Omega 3:

Omega-3s have important effects on basic lipid metabolism , they also have anti-inflammatory properties. These two properties gives them very varied, protective and curative effects on many pathologies.

- **Omega-3s and Inflammation-** All our cell membranes contain significant amounts of fatty acids. The more unsaturated the fat molecules, the more fluid the cell membrane and the easier the membrane exchange. This concept is of primary importance: a poorly fluid membrane will promote a chronic inflammatory state. Thus, a high level of DHA and EPA will produce a decrease in the inflammatory process. While the DHA provides especially good brain maintenance, the EPA (eicosapentaenoic acid) reduces inflammation (source of almost all age-related diseases), angiogenesis, blood pressure, atherosclerosis and triglycerides levels.

- **Omega-3s and Asthma-**Omega-3s reduce inflammation, a key component of asthma. They help improve lung function and reduce the amount of medication a person needs to control their condition.

- **Omega-3s and Joints-** Omega-3 (EPA / DHA) can reduce stiffness and joint pain. They also seem to increase the effectiveness of anti-inflammatory drugs. In addition, consuming omega-3s in addition to the drugs would slow the progression of rheumatoid arthritis, and therefore daily intake of omega-3s would increase the rates of remission and limit drug use.

- **Omega-3s and Obesity-** We know that being overweight can cause chronic inflammation of the body, but few people know that omega-3s can effectively lose weight and reduce the risk of cardiovascular disease. They even facilitate the burning of fat and thus protect the functional aspect of the cardiovascular system, and the aesthetic aspect by reducing overweight.

- **Omega-3s and Cholesterol and Triglycerides-** A majority of us are at risk of having a high level of harmful blood lipids. The proportions of good and bad cholesterol predispose or not to cardiovascular disease. Omega-3s help stabilize the relationship between good and bad cholesterol by making the ratio of bad cholesterol lower. They therefore lower the risk of atherosclerosis and coronary heart disease. Omega-3s can also reduce triglyceride levels, a plasmatic fat that, when found at high levels in the blood, is a significant risk factor for heart and digestive diseases.

- **Omega-3s and Diabetes-** It was already well known that omega-3s have positive effects on insulin resistance. In 2014, a natural molecule derived from omega-3 was discovered by researchers from Quebec affiliated with the Faculty of Medicine of Laval University. This molecule has beneficial effects on insulin resistance and treatment of type 2 diabetes and its effects are comparable to those of some drugs, including a hypoglycemic effect.

- **Omega-3s and Cardiovascular Diseases-** If omega-3 supplements are recommended for all, they are almost mandatory in case of heart risk. Their action on the heart is essential. Many studies prove it, omega-3s play a protective and fundamental role in the prevention of cardiovascular diseases. They prevent the formation of clots in the blood that can block blood vessels; they therefore reduce the risk of strokes (hemorrhagic or ischemic), heart failure and heart attacks.

- **Omega-3s and the Brain-** Lipids are essential to the normal functioning of the nervous system and more than 60% of our brain is fat composed mostly of docosahexaenoic acid (DHA).Omega-3s are the allies of the brain. They help fight depression, memory problems, Alzheimer's disease and Attention Deficit / Hyperactivity Disorder (ADHD). In addition, the DHA fraction is essential for membranes, synapses, mitochondria and the retina of the eye (they increase night vision). Many reports clearly show the benefits of omega-3s on the nervous system, which increase the number of neurotransmitters while ensuring proper brain function.

- **Omega-3s and Depression-** We have all experienced a little blues or a passing blunder. We now know that these bad mood states are often caused by an imbalance in omega-3s. More and more studies link mood swings to omega-3 deficiencies. Omega-3s are essential for emotional balance. They help fight against anxiety, stress and depression. Omega-3s EPA and DHA, once transformed in the body into prostaglandin derivatives, have anti-inflammatory properties. They facilitate the transmission of nerve impulses, and improve the growth and plasticity of nerve cells. Omega 3s may be a good alternative for patients who respond poorly to antidepressant drugs or who do not tolerate them, or for depressed people who refuse to take these drugs.

- **Omega-3s and Cognitive Functions-** Omega-3s can help protect brain function against dementia, memory loss and impaired cognitive abilities. The positive effect is considerable on the progressive memory loss associated with aging and the slowing progression of Alzheimer's disease. These effects are often linked to the fact that Omega-3s help the good transmission of nerve impulses and improve nerve cells plasticity. It should be noted that DHA (docosahexaenoic acid) is the major Omega-3 concerning effects on the nervous system.

- **Omega-3s and Gynecology-** Omega-3s are very important for the mom's mood stability and her well-being. During pregnancy and after delivery, they improve and facilitate the completion of pregnancy (Omega-3s and prostaglandins have linked metabolisms and therefore play a major role in the delivery process) and reduce the risk of postpartum depression. The consumption of omega-3s during pregnancy strengthens the immune system and reduces several health risks in the infant, such as allergies. They promote good psychomotor development, and especially for the nervous system and vision function of the future baby.

Characteristics of a high quality fish oil supplement

- Harvested from the ocean/sea

- Avoid fish oil from farm raised fish

- Pelagic fish to minimize environmental contaminations

- 3rd party tested for contamination, heavy metals, bacteria, fungi, impurities, etc.

- At least 500mg of actual omega-3 per serving

Dosage for Omega-3

Cardiovascular Benefits:

- Preventative dosage: 1000 mg total of EPA and DHA per day.

- Intervention (if you are already at risk of a cardiovascular condition): Up to 2000 mg total of EPA and DHA per day.

- Decrease inflammation: Between 2400 mg to 4000 mg total of EPA and DHA per day.

Nervous System/Psychological Benefits:

- Adolescent with ADHD (Attention Deficit Disorder with Hyperactivity): 2000 mg total of EPA and DHA with a minimum of 400 mg DHA per day.

- Depression: 4000 mg to 9000 mg total of EPA and DHA per day.

- Memory and cognitive decline: 3000 mg total of EPA and DHA, with a minimum of 1000 mg DHA per day.

***Disclaimer:** Again, please check with your health care provider before taking any supplements and/or changing your diet. The dosage mentioned in this book are general guidelines and are considered high dosages. Omega-3 fatty acids naturally have a blood thinning effect. This actually attributes to some of its cardiovascular benefits, but can cause side-effects for certain people. If you are on blood thinners, aspirin, and/or certain medications and supplements, please talk to your doctor before increasing omega-3/seafood consumption. Likewise, if you have a blood disorder, please let your primary doctor know before taking omega-3 fatty acids or increasing seafood consumption.

Supplements that fight inflammation:

- **Turmeric/Curcumin-** It is a component of the turmeric spice. It reduces inflammation in a wide range of diseases. It appears to be very beneficial for reducing inflammation and improving symptoms of osteoarthritis and rheumatoid arthritis (Panahi et al. 2016). A particular randomized controlled trial found out that people with metabolic syndrome who consumed curcumin had their levels of CRP and MDA (both inflammation markers) reduced compared to those who had a placebo (Panahi et al. 2015).

- **Ginger-** Ginger contains two important components – gingerol and zingerone. Both reduce inflammation linked to kidney damage, and colitis, breast cancer and diabetes (Rashidian et al. 2013)

- **Omega 3-** There are two active types of omega 3s – docosahexanoic acid and eicosapentanoic acid. Docosahexanoic acid in particular has potent anti-inflammatory effects that reduces the level of cytokines and promotes health of the gut. It also decreases muscle damage and inflammation that may occur after an exercise (Tabbaa et al. 2013).

- **Vitamin D3-** Recent research has shown the exact mechanism by which vitamin D3 inhibits inflammation. Vitamin D has a new receptor on DNA. When the vitamin binds on this receptor, then core gene signaling occurs that reduces inflammation. This is a very powerful anti-inflammatory mechanism. People that are deficient in vitamin D cannot activate this receptor, and are thus at high risk for inflammation (National Jewish Health, 2012).

REFRENCES:

1. Ward BW, Schiller JS, Goodman RA. Multiple chronic conditions among US adults: a 2012 update. Prev Chronic Dis. 2014;11:E62.

2. Centers for Disease Control and Prevention. Leading causes of death and numbers of deaths, by sex, race, and Hispanic origin: United States, 1980 and 2014 (Table 19). Health, United States, 2015. https://www.cdc.gov/nchs/data/hus/hus1 5.pdf#019[PDF – 13.4 MB]. Accessed June 21, 2017.

3. Ogden CL, Carroll MD, Fryar CD, Flegal KM. Prevalence of obesity among adults and youth: United States, 2011–2014. NCHS Data Brief. 2015 Nov ;(219):1-8.

4. Brault MW, Hootman J, Helmick CG, Theis KA, Armour BS. Prevalence and most common causes of disability among adults, United States, 2005. MMWR. 2009;58(16):421–426.

5. Barbour KE, Helmick CG, Boring M, Brady TJ. Prevalence of doctor-diagnosed arthritis and arthritis-attributable activity limitation—United States, 2013-2015. MMWR. 2017;66(9):246–253.

6. Centers for Disease Control and Prevention. National Diabetes Fact Sheet, 2011. http://www.cdc.gov/diabetes/pubs/pdf/ndfs_2011.pdf[PDF – 2.66 MB] Accessed December 20, 2013.

7. US Department of Health and Human Services. Healthy People 2020: Physical Activity. https://www.healthypeople.gov/2020/topics-objectives/topic/physical-activity/objectives. Accessed June 9, 2017.

8. Benjamin EJ, Blaha MJ, Chiuve SE, et al. Heart disease and stroke statistics—2017 update: a

report from the American Heart Association. Circulation. 2017;135:e1–e458.

9. Medzhitov, «Origin and Physiological Roles of Inflammation».

10. Seaman DR, Palombo AD. « An Overview of the Identification and Management of the Metabolic Syndrome in Chiropractic Practice.» in the Journal of Chiropractic Medicine. 2014;.

11. Leo Galland, MD. Diet and Inflammation.

12. Jun-Ming Zhang , and Jianxiong An, MSc, MD. Cytokines, Inflammation and Pain.

13. Lee et coll., «Impact of systemic inflammation on the relationship between insulin resistance and all-cause and cancer-related mortality», Metabolism Clinical and Experimental.

14. Balducci, S. et coll., «Anti-inflammatory effect of exercise training in subjects with type 2 diabetes and the metabolic syndrome is dependent on exercise modalities and independent of weight loss»,

15. World health organization official website: www.who.int/fr

16. National center of biotechnology information website: https://www.ncbi.nlm.nih.gov/

17. Barbara G, De Giorgio R, Stanghellini V, et al. A role for inflammation in irritable bowel syndrome? Gut 2002; 51:i41-i44.

18. Berk, M; Williams, L. J.; Jacka, F. N.; O'Neil, A; Pasco, J. A.; Moylan, S; Allen, N. B.; Stuart, A. L.; Hayley, A. C.; Byrne, M. L.; Maes, M (2013). "So depression is an inflammatory disease, but where does the inflammation come from?". BMC Medicine. 11: 200

19. Ferrero-Miliani L, Nielsen OH, Andersen PS, Girardin SE; Nielsen; Andersen; Girardin (2007). "Chronic inflammation: importance of NOD2 and NALP3 in interleukin-1beta generation". Clin. Exp. Immunol. 147 (2): 061127015327006

20. Golia E, Limongelli G, Natale F, Fimiani F, Maddaloni V, Pariggiano I, Bianchi R, Crisci M, D'Acierno L, Giordano R, Di Palma G, Conte M, Golino P, Russo MG, Calabrò R, Calabrò P. Inflammation and cardiovascular disease: from pathogenesis to therapeutic target. Curr Atheroscler Rep. 2014 Sep; 16(9):435.

21. Hall, John (2011). Guyton and Hall textbook of medical physiology (12th ed.). Philadelphia, Pa.: Saunders/Elsevier. p. 428. ISBN 978-1-4160-4574-8.

22. Hendrik Ungefroren; Susanne Sebens; Daniel Seidl; Hendrik Lehnert; Ralf Haas (2011). "Interaction of tumor cells with the microenvironment". Cell Communication and Signaling. 9 (18).

23. Libby, P (2002). "Inflammation in atherosclerosis". Nature. 420 (6917): 868–74.

24. National Jewish Health. (2012). How vitamin D inhibits inflammation. ScienceDaily. Retrieved June 26, 2018 from www.sciencedaily.com/releases/2012/02/120223 103920.htm

25. Panahi Y, Alishiri GH, Parvin S, Sahebkar A. Mitigation of Systemic Oxidative Stress by Curcuminoids in Osteoarthritis: Results of a Randomized Controlled Trial. J Diet Suppl. 2016; 13(2):209-20

26. Panahi Y, Hosseini MS, Khalili N, Naimi E, Majeed M, Sahebkar A. Antioxidant and anti-inflammatory effects of curcuminoid-piperine combination in subjects with metabolic syndrome: A randomized controlled trial and an updated meta-analysis. Clin Nutr. 2015 Dec; 34(6):1101-8

27. Rashidian A, Mehrzadi S, Ghannadi AR, Mahzooni P, Sadr S, Minaiyan M (2014).

Protective effect of ginger volatile oil against acetic acid-induced colitis in rats: a light microscopic evaluation. J Integr Med; 12(2):115-20.

28. Tabbaa, M., Golubic, M., Roizen, M. F., & Bernstein, A. M. (2013). Docosahexaenoic Acid, Inflammation, and Bacterial Dysbiosis in Relation to Periodontal Disease, Inflammatory Bowel Disease, and the Metabolic Syndrome. Nutrients, 5(8), 3299–3310. http://doi.org/10.3390/nu5083299

29. Wellen, K. E., & Hotamisligil, G. S. (2005). Inflammation, stress, and diabetes. Journal of Clinical Investigation, 115(5), 1111–1119. http://doi.org/10.1172/JCI200525102

30. Kodl CT, Seaquist ER: Cognitive dysfunction and diabetes mellitus. Endocr Rev 2008, 29:494-511.

31. Sommerfield AJ, Deary IJ, Frier BM: Acute hyperglycemia alters mood state and impairs cognitive performance in people with type 2 diabetes. Diabetes Care 2004, 27:2335-2340.

32. Ahmed SH, Guillem K, Vandaele Y: Sugar addiction: pushing the drug-sugar analogy to the limit. Curr Opin Clin Nutr Metab Care 2013, 16:434-439.

33. Lenoir M, Serre F, Cantin L, et al: Intense sweetness surpasses cocaine reward. PLoS One 2007, 2:e698.

34. Lennerz BS, Alsop DC, Holsen LM, et al: Effects of dietary glycemic index on brain regions related to reward and craving in men. Am J Clin Nutr 2013.

35. The World Health Organization official website: www.who.int

36. National Center for Biotechnology Information website: www.ncbi.nlm.nih.gov

37. Schmidt MA: Brain-Building Nutrition. Frog, California, 1997.

38. Lombard J; Willner C,: Neuroprotection, a Functional Medecine Approach for Common and Uncommon Neurologic Syndromes, Washington, Institute for Fonctional Medecine, 2005.

39. Bland JS: Understanding the Origins and Applying Advanced Nutritional Strategies for Autoimmune Diseases. Metagenics inc., 2006-11-11.

40. https://www.webmd.com/vitamins/ai/ingredient mono-662/turmeric

41. National cancer institute official website: https://www.cancer.gov/publications/dictionaries/cancer-drug/def/curcumin.

Systemic Gluten Sensitivity Checklist- circle any of the relevant symptoms on the 0-10 scale, with 10 being very severe symptoms and 0 being not symptomatic at all.

Today's Date: ______________________

1.	Headaches	0-1-2-3-4-5-6-7-8-9-10
2.	Fatigue	0-1-2-3-4-5-6-7-8-9-10
3.	Brain Fog	0-1-2-3-4-5-6-7-8-9-10
4.	Depression	0-1-2-3-4-5-6-7-8-9-10
5.	Thyroid Dysfunction	0-1-2-3-4-5-6-7-8-9-10
6.	Bloating	0-1-2-3-4-5-6-7-8-9-10
7.	Stomach Discomfort	0-1-2-3-4-5-6-7-8-9-10
8.	Skin Rash/Itchiness	0-1-2-3-4-5-6-7-8-9-10
9.	Painful Menses	0-1-2-3-4-5-6-7-8-9-10
10.	Achy Muscles/Joints	0-1-2-3-4-5-6-7-8-9-10

***Score:** ______________

*Now add all the numbers that you have circled together and write the sum above in the "Score" section. You can think of this as your current gluten sensitivity score. I have included the exact same test again at the end of the book, so that you can compare your score from before and after you complete the 30 day gluten free challenge.

Systemic Gluten Sensitivity Checklist- circle any of the relevant symptoms on the 0-10 scale, with 10 being very severe symptoms and 0 being not symptomatic at all.

Today's Date: ______________________

1.	Headaches	0-1-2-3-4-5-6-7-8-9-10
2.	Fatigue	0-1-2-3-4-5-6-7-8-9-10
3.	Brain Fog	0-1-2-3-4-5-6-7-8-9-10
4.	Depression	0-1-2-3-4-5-6-7-8-9-10
5.	Thyroid Dysfunction	0-1-2-3-4-5-6-7-8-9-10
6.	Bloating	0-1-2-3-4-5-6-7-8-9-10
7.	Stomach Discomfort	0-1-2-3-4-5-6-7-8-9-10
8.	Skin Rash/Itchiness	0-1-2-3-4-5-6-7-8-9-10
9.	Painful Menses	0-1-2-3-4-5-6-7-8-9-10
10.	Achy Muscles/Joints	0-1-2-3-4-5-6-7-8-9-10

***Score:** ______________

*Now add all the numbers that you have circled together and write the sum above in the "Score" section. You can think of this as your current gluten sensitivity score. I have included the exact same test again at the end of the book, so that you can compare your score from before and after you complete the 30 day gluten free challenge.

Systemic Gluten Sensitivity Checklist- circle any of the relevant symptoms on the 0-10 scale, with 10 being very severe symptoms and 0 being not symptomatic at all.

Today's Date: ___________________________

1. Headaches   0-1-2-3-4-5-6-7-8-9-10
2. Fatigue   0-1-2-3-4-5-6-7-8-9-10
3. Brain Fog   0-1-2-3-4-5-6-7-8-9-10
4. Depression   0-1-2-3-4-5-6-7-8-9-10
5. Thyroid Dysfunction   0-1-2-3-4-5-6-7-8-9-10
6. Bloating   0-1-2-3-4-5-6-7-8-9-10
7. Stomach Discomfort   0-1-2-3-4-5-6-7-8-9-10
8. Skin Rash/Itchiness   0-1-2-3-4-5-6-7-8-9-10
9. Painful Menses   0-1-2-3-4-5-6-7-8-9-10
10. Achy Muscles/Joints   0-1-2-3-4-5-6-7-8-9-10

***Score:** _____________

*Now add all the numbers that you have circled together and write the sum above in the "Score" section. You can think of this as your current gluten sensitivity score. I have included the exact same test again at the end of the book, so that you can compare your score from before and after you complete the 30 day gluten free challenge.

ABOUT THE AUTHOR

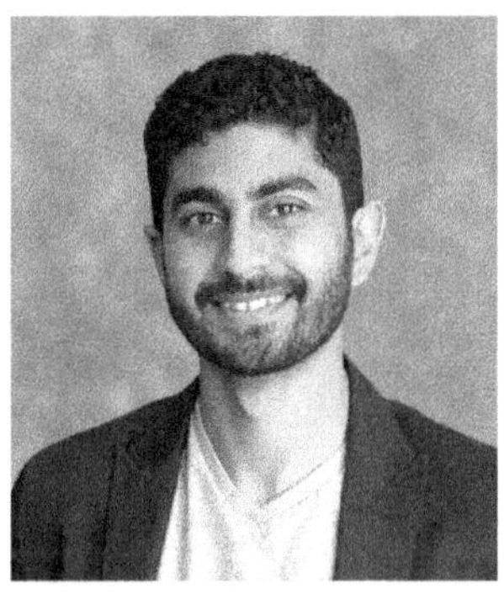

Due to his leadership and achievements in wholistic healing, Dr. Mina Botros was recognized as one of the **"Leading Physicians of the World"** and **Top Doctor** in his field by **"The International Association of Healthcare Professionals"**. You may recognize Dr. Mina Botros from:

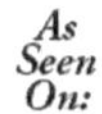

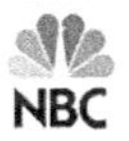
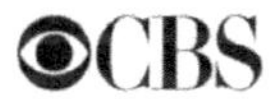
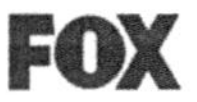

Dr. Mina always knew it was his calling to help other people reach their goals, largely through health and wellbeing. For him, this initially meant an interest in psychiatry, understanding the human mind, motivation and behaviors. It wasn't until he'd completed his psychology and pre-med degree at the University of Wisconsin-

Milwaukee that his perspective began to change. "I realized that the standard health model is wonderful for treating many severe cases—heart attacks, infections, ruptures and organ failures—but it did a very poor job preventing them in the first place," he says. "I didn't like the idea that we have to wait till a problem arises to treat it."

Dr. Mina genuinely believed, and still does, that health isn't a destination but a journey, and that we can all live a healthy, fulfilling lifestyle if we learn how to prevent instead of "fix." This realization led him to a decision; he didn't want to be a doctor that treats the problem after it's too late. He wanted to be the doctor that detects the root cause of an issue as soon as it manifests, treating it right away. After doing some research, he found chiropractic—a way he could help people feel better, get healthier and find results without drugs or surgery.

In practice, it's Dr. Mina's personal mission to be the bridge that brings people from where they are now to where they want to be. "I think that we all need to live a life we are proud of," he says. "Everyone has a definition of that, and that is what makes this world so beautiful and colorful." As a healer, he aims to help fuel that beauty and color by making sure his patients feel and function their best. This way, they have nothing holding them back from living their happiest, most authentic lives.

In his free time, Dr. Mina loves camping, hiking, stargazing and cooking Mediterranean food. He really enjoys ending a good, productive day playing board games with his friends, having meaningful conversation and sharing a meal together. His favorite quote is **"Create the life you dream of"** which for him embodies a message of hope, possibility and faith.